50 Studies Every Urologist Should Know

50 STUDIES EVERY DOCTOR SHOULD KNOW

50 Studies Every Doctor Should Know: The Key Studies that Form the Foundation of Evidence Based Medicine, Revised Edition
Michael E. Hochman

50 Studies Every Internist Should Know
Kristopher Swiger, Joshua R. Thomas, Michael E. Hochman, and Steven Hochman

50 Studies Every Neurologist Should Know
David Y. Hwang and David M. Greer

50 Studies Every Pediatrician Should Know
Ashaunta T. Anderson, Nina L. Shapiro, Stephen C. Aronoff, Jeremiah Davis, and Michael Levy

50 Imaging Studies Every Doctor Should Know
Christoph I. Lee

50 Studies Every Surgeon Should Know
SreyRam Kuy, Rachel J. Kwon, and Miguel A. Burch

50 Studies Every Intensivist Should Know
Edward A. Bittner

50 Studies Every Palliative Care Doctor Should Know
David Hui, Akhila Reddy, and Eduardo Bruera

50 Studies Every Psychiatrist Should Know
Ish P. Bhalla, Rajesh R. Tampi, and Vinod H. Srihari

50 Studies Every Anesthesiologist Should Know
Anita Gupta, Michael E. Hochman, and Elena N. Gutman

50 Studies Every Ophthalmologist Should Know
Alan D. Penman, Kimberly W. Crowder, and William M. Watkins, Jr.

50 Studies Every Urologist Should Know
Philipp Dahm

50 Studies Every Urologist Should Know

EDITED BY

PHILIPP DAHM, MD, MHSc

Professor of Urology
University of Minnesota
Urology Vice-Chair of Education and Program Director
Director of Specialty Care/Surgery Research
Minneapolis VAMC
St. Paul, MN, USA

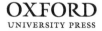

OXFORD
UNIVERSITY PRESS

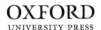

Oxford University Press is a department of the University of Oxford. It furthers the University's objective of excellence in research, scholarship, and education by publishing worldwide. Oxford is a registered trade mark of Oxford University Press in the UK and certain other countries.

Published in the United States of America by Oxford University Press
198 Madison Avenue, New York, NY 10016, United States of America.

Library of Congress Cataloging-in-Publication Data
Names: Dahm, Philipp, editor.
Title: 50 studies every urologist should know / [edited by] Philipp Dahm.
Other titles: Fifty studies every urologist should know | 50 studies every doctor should know (Series)
Description: New York, NY : Oxford University Press, [2021] |
Series: 50 studies every doctor should know | Includes bibliographical references and index.
Identifiers: LCCN 2021000934 (print) | LCCN 2021000935 (ebook) |
ISBN 9780190655341 (paperback) | ISBN 9780190655365 (epub) |
ISBN 9780190655372 (online)
Subjects: MESH: Urologic Diseases | Prostatic Diseases |
Evidence-Based Medicine | Clinical Trials as Topic
Classification: LCC RC871 (print) | LCC RC871 (ebook) |
NLM WJ 140 | DDC 616.6—dc23
LC record available at https://lccn.loc.gov/2021000934
LC ebook record available at https://lccn.loc.gov/2021000935

DOI: 10.1093/med/9780190655341.001.0001

9 8 7 6 5 4 3 2 1

Printed by Marquis, Canada

CONTENTS

Foreword xi
Preface from the Series Editor xiii
Contributors xv

1. Early Detection of Prostate Cancer: The European Randomized Study of Screening for Prostate Cancer (ERSPC) 1
   Philipp Dahm

2. The Influence of Finasteride on the Development of Prostate Cancer: Prostate Cancer Prevention Trial (PCPT) 7
   Niranjan Sathianathen

3. MRI-Targeted or Standard Biopsy for Prostate Cancer Diagnosis: The PRECISION Trial 13
   Philipp Dahm

4. Long-Term Survival Among Men With Conservatively Treated Localized Prostate Cancer: Conservative Management of Prostate Cancer 19
   Niranjan Sathianathen and Philipp Dahm

5. Clinical Results of Long-Term Follow-Up of a Large, Active Surveillance Cohort With Localized Prostate Cancer 25
   Niranjan Sathianathen

6. Radical Prostatectomy Versus Observation in Early Prostate Cancer: Scandinavian Prostate Cancer Group Study Number 4 (SPCG-4) 31
   Philipp Dahm

7. Radical Prostatectomy Versus Observation for Localized Prostate
   Cancer: The Prostate Cancer Intervention Versus Observation
   Trial (PIVOT) 37
   Philipp Dahm

8. 10-Year Outcomes After Monitoring, Surgery, or Radiotherapy:
   The Prostate Testing for Cancer and Treatment (ProtecT) Trial 43
   Philipp Dahm

9. Comparative Effectiveness of Minimally Invasive Versus Open Radical
   Prostatectomy 49
   Philipp Dahm

10. Quality of Life and Satisfaction With Outcome Among Prostate Cancer
    Survivors: Quality of Life After Primary Treatment of Localized Prostate
    Cancer 55
    Niranjan Sathianathen and Philipp Dahm

11. Adjuvant Radiotherapy for Pathologically Advanced Prostate Cancer:
    A Southwest Oncology Group Randomized Controlled Trial
    (SWOG 8794) 61
    Philipp Dahm

12. Survival Following Primary Androgen Deprivation Therapy Among
    Men With Localized Prostate Cancer 67
    Joseph Zabell

13. Bilateral Orchiectomy With or Without Flutamide for Metastatic
    Prostate Cancer 73
    Philipp Dahm

14. Intermittent Versus Continuous Androgen Deprivation in Prostate
    Cancer: Intermittent Androgen Deprivation Therapy (SWOG Trial
    9346) 77
    Niranjan Sathianathen and Philipp Dahm

15. Docetaxel Plus Prednisone or Mitoxantrone Plus Prednisone for
    Advanced Prostate Cancer: The TAX 327 Trial 83
    Joseph Zabell

16. Chemohormonal Therapy in Metastatic Hormone-Sensitive Prostate
    Cancer: The Chemohormonal Therapy Versus Androgen Ablation
    Randomized Trial for Extensive Disease in Prostate Cancer
    (CHAARTED) Trial 89
    Philipp Dahm

17. Abiraterone and Increased Survival in Metastatic Prostate Cancer 95
Joseph Zabell

18. Enzalutamide in Metastatic Prostate Cancer Before Chemotherapy:
The PREVAIL Study 101
Joseph Zabell

19. The EORTC Intergroup Phase 3 Study Comparing the Oncological
Outcome of Elective Nephron-Sparing Surgery and Radical
Nephrectomy for Low-Stage Renal Cell Carcinoma 107
Christopher Weight

20. Nephrectomy Followed by Interferon Alfa-2b Compared With
Interferon Alfa-2b Alone for Metastatic Renal Cell Cancer 113
Christopher Weight

21. Sunitinib Versus Interferon Alfa in Metastatic Renal Cell Carcinoma 119
Christopher Weight

22. Nivolumab Versus Everolimus in Advanced Renal Cell
Carcinoma: CheckMate 025 123
Christopher Weight

23. The Effect of Intravesical Mitomycin C on Recurrence of Newly
Diagnosed Superficial Bladder Cancer: A Further Report
With 7 Years of Follow-Up 129
Vikram M. Narayan

24. Bacillus Calmette–Guérin (BCG) Immunotherapy for Recurrent
Noninvasive Transitional Cell Carcinoma of the Bladder: A Randomized
Southwest Oncology Group (SWOG) Study 135
Vikram M. Narayan

25. Neoadjuvant Chemotherapy Plus Cystectomy Compared With
Cystectomy Alone for Locally Advanced Bladder Cancer 141
Vikram M. Narayan

26. Radiotherapy With or Without Chemotherapy in Muscle-Invasive
Bladder Cancer 147
Vikram M. Narayan

27. A Randomized Comparison of Cisplatin Alone or in Combination With
Methotrexate, Vinblastine, and Doxorubicin in Patients With Metastatic
Urothelial Carcinoma: A Cooperative Group Study 153
Philipp Dahm and Vikram M. Narayan

28. Gemcitabine and Cisplatin Versus Methotrexate, Vinblastine, Doxorubicin, and Cisplatin in Advanced or Metastatic Bladder Cancer: Results of a Large, Randomized, Multinational, Multicenter, Phase III Study 159
Vikram M. Narayan

29. Pembrolizumab as Second-Line Therapy for Advanced Urothelial Carcinoma: KEYNOTE-045 165
Philipp Dahm and Vikram M. Narayan

30. Cis-Diamminedichloroplatinum, Vinblastine, and Bleomycin Combination Chemotherapy in Disseminated Testicular Cancer 171
Michael Risk

31. Treatment of Disseminated Germ Cell Tumors With Cisplatin, Bleomycin, and Either Vinblastine or Etoposide: PVB Versus BEP 177
Michael Risk

32. Urinary Volume, Water Intake, and Stone Recurrence in Idiopathic Calcium Nephrolithiasis: A 5-Year Randomized Prospective Study 183
Michael S. Borofsky and Vincent G. Bird

33. A Prospective Study of Dietary Calcium and Other Nutrients and the Risk of Symptomatic Kidney Stones 189
Michael S. Borofsky and Vincent G. Bird

34. First Clinical Experience With Extracorporeally Induced Destruction of Kidney Stones by Shock Waves 193
Michael S. Borofsky and Vincent G. Bird

35. Shock Wave Lithotripsy Versus Ureteroscopy for Lower-Pole Caliceal Calculi 1 cm or Less 197
Vincent G. Bird and Michael S. Borofsky

36. Extracorporeal Shock Wave Lithotripsy Versus Percutaneous Nephrolithotomy for Lower-Pole Nephrolithiasis: The Lower Pole I Study 203
Vincent G. Bird and Michael S. Borofsky

37. Medical Expulsive Therapy (MET) in Adults With Ureteric Colic: The Spontaneous Urinary Stone Passage Enabled by Drugs (SUSPEND) Trial 209
Michael S. Borofsky and Vincent G. Bird

38. Burch Colposuspension Versus Fascial Sling to Reduce Urinary Stress Incontinence: The Stress Incontinence Surgical Treatment Efficacy (SISTEr) Trial 215
   Colby A. Dixon, Giulia I. Lane, Cynthia S. Fok, and M. Louis Moy

39. Retropubic Versus Transobturator Midurethral Slings for Stress Incontinence: The Trial of Mid Urethral Slings (TOMUS) 221
   Giulia I. Lane, Colby A. Dixon, M. Louis Moy, and Cynthia S. Fok

40. A Midurethral Sling to Reduce Incontinence After Vaginal Prolapse Repair: The Outcomes Following Vaginal Prolapse Repair and Midurethral Sling (OPUS) Trial 227
   Giulia I. Lane, Colby A. Dixon, M. Louis Moy, and Cynthia S. Fok

41. A Randomized Trial of Urodynamic Testing Before Stress Incontinence Surgery: The Value of Urodynamic Evaluation (ValUE) Trial 233
   Colby A. Dixon, Giulia I. Lane, Cynthia S. Fok, and M. Louis Moy

42. Anticholinergic Therapy Versus Onabotulinumtoxin A for Urgency Urinary Incontinence: The Anticholinergic Versus Botulinum Toxin Comparison (ABC) Study 239
   Giulia I. Lane, Colby A. Dixon, M. Louis Moy, and Cynthia S. Fok

43. Oral Sildenafil in the Treatment of Erectile Dysfunction 245
   Joshua Bodie

44. Treatment of Men With Erectile Dysfunction With Transurethral Alprostadil 251
   Joshua Bodie

45. Antimicrobial Prophylaxis for Children With Vesicoureteral Reflux: Randomized Intervention for Children With Vesicoureteral Reflux (RIVUR) Trial 257
   Philipp Dahm and Jane M. Lewis

46. A Comparison of Transurethral Surgery With Watchful Waiting for Moderate Symptoms of Benign Prostatic Hyperplasia: The Veterans Affairs Cooperative Study Group on Transurethral Resection of the Prostate 263
   Jae Hung Jung

47. The Efficacy of Terazosin, Finasteride, or Both in Benign Prostatic Hyperplasia: The Veterans Affairs Cooperative Benign Prostatic Hyperplasia Study 269
   Jae Hung Jung

48. Chlorhexidine–Alcohol Versus Povidone–Iodine for Surgical-Site
    Antisepsis 275
    Philipp Dahm

49. Clean Intermittent Self-Catheterization in the Treatment of Urinary Tract
    Disease 281
    Jeffrey I. Estrin and Sean P. Elliott

50. The Surgical Learning Curve for Prostate Cancer Control After Radical
    Prostatectomy 287
    Philipp Dahm

Index 293

FOREWORD

Starting with training and during my academic career in urology, I was often faced with a quandary regarding how to identify and cull out the most significant literature. I felt this would enable me to recall data from specific publications which I could use in a particular clinical situation. I daresay many of you have faced a similar quandary at some point. I am certain many of us are familiar with a few of the "landmark" publications that are often cited by various teachers, peers, and accomplished academicians. Given the rate at which literature is being generated today (>900,000 citations added to PubMed each year), one can get lost in this information deluge without being able to recognize what papers are most practice changing. It is important for trainees and practitioners to be aware of the key publications which shaped the practice of urology and have these papers available as a ready reference. This allows for subsequent reexamination of the original data in the context of new information or in the context of a particular case. It also allows one to identify gaps highlighted by prior studies that can spur new research. Being able to personally review the source citations also allows the individual practitioner to analyze the study structure and validity of the results and understand the limitations presented by the data which can inform how they are applied in practice.

With increasing understanding of the nuances of study design and statistical evaluation, one can determine how pertinent and valid the data from these "landmark" studies is and whether it is still pertinent. *50 Studies Every Urologist Should Know* is a remarkable and invaluable compendium of the key "gold standard" literature in urology. This book is a painstakingly curated assembly of the most impactful published literature in urology over the past nearly five decades. There are sections on each of the urologic cancers, stone disease, female urology, LUTS, pediatric urology, and erectile dysfunction. It will serve as a ready reference for individuals caring for urologic patients at all levels. The particularly unique feature of the book is that each study is described in detail and individually explained and critiqued by experts in the field. The study schema and the salient findings are described very succinctly and are easy to grasp. References to other relevant studies are included, as well as patient examples to illustrate how one would apply the data from the studies into clinical practice. Hence this compendium would serve as an interpretive guide to the published papers themselves. I find this book to be a must-have addition to my academic library and I sincerely believe you will find it to be just as useful.

Enjoy reading,

Badrinath R. Konety, MBBS, MBA
Dean of Rush Medical College and
Senior Vice President of Clinical Affairs for
Rush University System
Chicago, IL, USA

PREFACE FROM THE SERIES EDITOR

When I was a third-year medical student, I asked one of my senior residents—who seemed to be able to quote every medical study in the history of mankind—if he had a list of key studies that have defined the current practice of general medicine that I should read before graduating medical school. "Don't worry," he told me. "You will learn the key studies as you go along."

But picking up on these key studies didn't prove so easy, and I was frequently admonished by my attendings for being unaware of crucial literature in their field. More importantly, because I had a mediocre understanding of the medical literature at that time, I lacked confidence in my clinical decision-making and had difficulty appreciating the significance of new research findings. It wasn't until I was well into my residency—thanks to a considerable amount of effort and determination—that I finally began to feel comfortable with both the emerging and fundamental medical literature.

Now, as a practicing general internist, I realize that I am not the only doctor who has struggled to become familiar with the key medical studies that form the foundation of evidence-based practice. Many of the students and residents I work with tell me that they feel overwhelmed by the medical literature, and that they cannot process new research findings because they lack a solid understanding of what has already been published. Even many practicing physicians—including those with years of experience—have only a cursory knowledge of the medical evidence base and make clinical decisions largely on personal experience.

I initially wrote *50 Studies Every Doctor Should Know* in an attempt to provide medical professionals (and even lay readers interested in learning more about medical research) a quick way to get up to speed on the classic studies that shape clinical practice. But it soon became clear there was a greater need for this distillation of the medical evidence than my original book provided. Soon after the book's publication, I began receiving calls from specialist physicians in a variety of disciplines wondering about the possibility of another book focusing on studies in their field. In partnership with a wonderful team of editors from Oxford University Press, we have developed my initial book into a series, offering volumes in Internal Medicine, Pediatrics, Surgery, Neurology, Radiology, Critical Care, Anesthesia, Psychiatry, Palliative Care, Ophthalmology, and now Urology. Several additional volumes are in the works.

I am excited about this latest volume in Urology, which is the culmination of hard work by the editor, Philipp Dahm, who has summarized the most important studies in his field. Particularly over the past several years, there has become a solid evidence based in the field of Urology, and Dr. Dahm has effectively captured it in this volume. I believe *50 Studies Every Urologist Should Know* provides the perfect launching ground for trainees in the field as well as a helpful refresher for practicing physicians and clinicians in the field. The book also highlights key knowledge gaps that may stimulate researchers to tackle key unanswered questions in the field. A special thanks also goes to the wonderful editors at Oxford University Press—Marta Moldvai and Tiffany Lu—who injected energy and creativity into the production process for this volume. This volume was a pleasure to help develop, and I learned a lot about the field of Urology in the process.

I have no doubt you will gain important insights into the field of Urology in the pages ahead!

Michael E. Hochman, MD, MPH

CONTRIBUTORS

Vincent G. Bird, MD
David A. Cofrin Endowed Professor
   of Urology
Chief, Division of Minimally
   Invasive Surgery
Endourology/Minimally
   Invasive Surgery Fellowship
   Co-Director
Department of Urology
University of Florida College of
   Medicine
Gainesville, FL, USA

Joshua Bodie, MD
Associate Professor
Department of Urology
University of Minnesota
Arden Hills, MN, USA

Michael S. Borofsky, MD
Assistant Professor
Department of Urology
University of Minnesota
Minneapolis, MN, USA

Philipp Dahm, MD, MHSc
Professor of Urology
University of Minnesota
Urology Vice-Chair of Education and
   Program Director
Director of Specialty Care/Surgery
   Research
Minneapolis VAMC
St. Paul, MN, USA

Colby A. Dixon, MD
Department of Urology
HealthPartners Specialty Center
St. Paul, MN, USA

Sean P. Elliott, MD, MS
Cloverfields Professor and Vice Chair
   of Urology
University of Minnesota
Minneapolis, MN, USA

Jeffrey I. Estrin, MS, PA-C
Physician Assistant
Department of Urology
Hennepin Healthcare
Minneapolis, MN, USA

Cynthia S. Fok, MD, MPH
Assistant Professor
Department of Urology
University of Minnesota
Minneapolis, MN, USA

Jae Hung Jung, MD, PhD
Professor
Department of Urology
Yonsei University Wonju College
  of Medicine
Wonju, Gangwon, Republic
  of Korea

Giulia I. Lane, MD, MS
Urologist
Department of Urology
University of Michigan
Ann Arbor, MI, USA

Jane M. Lewis, MD
Associate Professor
Department of Urology
University of Minnesota
Minneapolis, MN, USA

M. Louis Moy, MD
Associate Professor of Urology
Department of Urology
University of Florida
Gainesville, FL, USA

Vikram M. Narayan, MD
Assistant Professor
Department of Urology
Emory University School of Medicine
Director of Urologic Oncology
Grady Memorial Hospital
Atlanta, GA, USA

Michael Risk, MD, PhD
Associate Professor
Department of Urology
University of Minnesota
Minneapolis, MN, USA

**Niranjan Sathianathen, MBBS
(Hons), PGDipSurgAnat,
PGDipSurgSci**
Urology Registrar
University of Melbourne
Flemington, VI, Australia

Christopher Weight, MD, MS
Glickman Urologic and Kidney Institute
Cleveland Clinic
Waite Hill, OH, USA

Joseph Zabell, MD
Assistant Professor
Department of Urology
University of Minnesota
Minneapolis, MN, USA

1

Early Detection of Prostate Cancer

The European Randomized Study of Screening for Prostate Cancer (ERSPC)

PHILIPP DAHM

"PSA-based screening reduced the rate of death from prostate cancer by 20% but was associated with a high risk of overdiagnosis."[1]

Research Question: In men at risk for prostate cancer, does prostate-specific antigen (PSA) screening compared to no screening reduce prostate cancer mortality?

Funding: Several sources, including Europe Against Cancer, the fifth and sixth framework program of the European Union, Beckman Coulter, as well as several local grants.

Year Study Began: June 1991 (study start varied substantially by European country)

Year Study Published: March 2009

Study Location: National study centers representing nine countries (The Netherlands, Belgium, Sweden, Finland, Italy, Spain, Switzerland, France, and

Portugal); of these, Portugal discontinued participation and France only joined in 2001 so did not have mature data at initial time of publication.

Who Was Studied: Men ages 50 to 74 years

Who Was Excluded: Men with a past or current history of prostate cancer

Patients: 182,160

Study Overview:

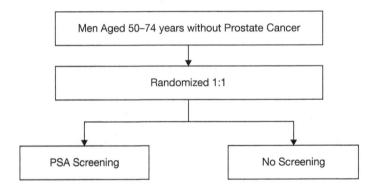

Study Interventions: Eligible men were identified through population registries. Recruitment and randomization procedures differed among countries. In some countries men in the screening arms were randomized before consenting, in others after consenting. Men in the no-screening arms were consistently not consented. The most common screening interval was 4 years (range 2 to 7 years) and 3 ng/ml was the most commonly used threshold for recommending a biopsy.

Follow-up: Median follow-up of approximately 9 years

Endpoints: Primary outcome: prostate-cancer mortality. Secondary outcomes: complications, progression-free (tumor-free) survival, survival free of metastasis, serious side effects of the screening procedure and of treatment, quality of life.

RESULTS:

- The mean age at randomization was 60.8 years (range: 59.6 to 63.0).
- In the screening arm, 82.2% of men were screened at least once; each man had an average of 2.1 PSA tests.
- 16.2% of PSA tests were "positive"; the average rate of compliance with a biopsy recommendation was 85.8%.
- Of men undergoing a biopsy for an elevated PSA, the false-positive rate was 75.9%.
- 5,990 men (8.2%) were diagnosed with prostate cancer in the screening group compared to 4307 (4.8%) in the no-screening group.
- There were 214 prostate cancer deaths in the screening group and 326 in the control group; the rate ratio for dying from prostate cancer was 0.80 (95% confidence interval [CI], 0.67 to 0.95).
- The corresponding number to screen was 1,410 (95% CI, 1,142 to 1,721).

Criticism and Limitations: The fact that men in the screening arm but not the no-screening arm were consented may have been a source of prognostic imbalance. Also, there was considerable heterogeneity within the trial with regard to the intervention. It provides little direct evidence on the downstream treatment-related harms. Minority enrollment was negligible. Nevertheless, this study is regarded as providing the highest quality of evidence on the effects of PSA screening.[2]

Other Relevant Studies and Information:

- Updates of this trial with follow-up of 16 years including men enrolled in the French study arm have since been reported. The rate ratio was 0.80 (95% CI, 0.72 to 0.89); the resulting number-needed-to-be-invited for screening to prevent one additional death from prostate cancer was 570.[2]
- The Prostate, Lung, Colon, and Ovarian (PLCO) Cancer Screening Trial was published around the same time and did not demonstrate a mortality benefit of screening. However, it has been criticized for high rates of contamination in the no-screening arm.[3]
- A primary-care–based, cluster randomized controlled trial randomized 419,582 men to a single PSA test versus no screening and found no reduction of mortality.[4]

- Current evidence-based guidelines on PSA screening vary considerably[5–7] but generally agree on the imperative of shared decision making. The US Preventive Services Task Force has issued a grade C recommendation against PSA screening in men aged 55 to 69 and a grade D recommendation against PSA screening in men 70 years or older.[8]

Summary and Implications: ERSPC provides the most methodologically rigorous study of the potential benefits and harms of prostate cancer screening and therefore commands a special place in systematic reviews supporting current evidence-based guidelines.[2, 9,10] Its findings indicate a small mortality benefit of PSA screening that needs to be weighed against the risk of overdiagnosis and overtreatment.

CLINICAL CASE: PSA SCREENING

Case History:

A 74-year-old patient is seen in the urology practice for a symptomatic ureteral stone and undergoes ureteroscopic laser stone fragmentation following unsuccessful medical expulsive therapy. He has a past medical history of hypertension, coronary artery disease, and mild chronic obstructive pulmonary disease. He has no family history of prostate cancer and has not undergone prior PSA testing or a biopsy. He asks whether he should have a PSA test done for early detection of prostate cancer.

Suggested Answer:

The patient's presentation is notable for an age of 74 years and substantial medical comorbidities. The results of the ERSPC trial indicate that this patient may derive a small survival benefit in terms of prostate-cancer–specific mortality (not all-cause mortality). Such a benefit is most likely realized in men with an extended life expectancy of 15 years or greater. The potential harms of PSA-based prostate cancer screening include a high rate of false-positive tests, biopsy-related complications, the unnecessary diagnosis of low-risk prostate cancer unlikely to affect a man during his lifetime (overdiagnosis) in some, and treatment sequelae both in men who may benefit from treatment and those who will not (overtreatment). Whereas the decision to have a PSA test is a very personal one that a well-informed patient should make based on his own values and preferences, this man appears unlikely to benefit from PSA testing.

References

1. Schroder FH, Hugosson J, Roobol MJ, et al. Screening and prostate-cancer mortality in a randomized European study. *N Engl J Med* 2009;360(13):1320–8. doi: 10.1056/NEJMoa0810084

2. Ilic D, Djulbegovic M, Jung JH, et al. Prostate cancer screening with prostate-specific antigen (PSA) test: a systematic review and meta-analysis. *BMJ* 2018;362:k3519. doi: 10.1136/bmj.k3519 [published online first: 2018/09/07]

3. Shoag JE, Mittal S, Hu JC. Reevaluating PSA testing rates in the PLCO trial. *N Engl J Med* 2016;374(18):1795–6. doi: 10.1056/NEJMc1515131 [published online first: 2016/05/06]

4. Martin RM, Donovan JL, Turner EL, et al. Effect of a low-intensity PSA-based screening intervention on prostate cancer mortality: the CAP randomized clinical trial. *JAMA* 2018;319(9):883–95. doi: 10.1001/jama.2018.0154 [published online first: 2018/03/07]

5. Carter HB, Albertsen PC, Barry MJ, et al. Early detection of prostate cancer: AUA guideline. *J Urol* 2013;190(2):419–26. doi: 10.1016/j.juro.2013.04.119 [published online first: 2013/05/11]

6. Mottet N, Bellmunt J, Bolla M, et al. EAU-ESTRO-SIOG guidelines on prostate cancer. Part 1: screening, diagnosis, and local treatment with curative intent. *Eur Urol* 2017;71(4):618–29. doi: 10.1016/j.eururo.2016.08.003 [published online first: 2016/08/30]

7. Tikkinen KAO, Dahm P, Lytvyn L, et al. Prostate cancer screening with prostate-specific antigen (PSA) test: a clinical practice guideline. *BMJ* 2018;362:k3581. doi: 10.1136/bmj.k3581 [published online first: 2018/09/07]

8. US Preventive Services Task Force, Grossman DC, Curry SJ, et al. Screening for prostate cancer: US Preventive Services Task Force recommendation statement. *JAMA* 2018;319(18):1901–13. doi: 10.1001/jama.2018.3710 [published online first: 2018/05/26]

9. Ilic D, Neuberger MM, Djulbegovic M, et al. Screening for prostate cancer. *Cochrane Database Syst Rev* 2013;(1):CD004720. doi: 10.1002/14651858.CD004720.pub3 [published online first: 2013/02/27]

10. Fenton JJ, Weyrich MS, Durbin S, et al. Prostate-specific antigen-based screening for prostate cancer: evidence report and systematic review for the US Preventive Services Task Force. *JAMA* 2018;319(18):1914–31. doi: 10.1001/jama.2018.3712 [published online first: 2018/05/26]

2

The Influence of Finasteride on the Development of Prostate Cancer

Prostate Cancer Prevention Trial (PCPT)

NIRANJAN SATHIANATHEN

"Finasteride prevents or delays the appearance of prostate cancer, but this possible benefit and a reduced risk of urinary problems must be weighed against sexual side effects and the increased risk of high-grade prostate cancer."[1]

Research Question: In men over the age of 55 years with a normal digital rectal examination (DRE) and a low prostate-specific antigen (PSA; 3.0 ng/ml or less), does treatment with finasteride reduce the risk of prostate cancer development?

Funding: Merck provided the finasteride and the placebo; trial was supported in part by Public Health Service grants from the National Cancer Institute.

Year Study Began: 1994

Year Study Published: 2003

Study Location: Multicenter, United States

Who Was Studied: Men over the age of 55 years with a normal DRE, a PSA of 3.0 ng/ml or less, no clinically significant coexisting conditions, and an American Urological Association symptom score of less than 20

Who Was Excluded: Men with a PSA of more than 3.0 ng/ml

Patients: 18,882

Study Overview:

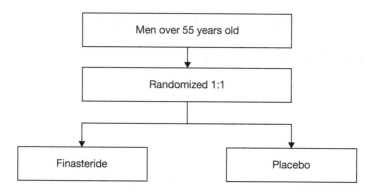

Study Interventions: Eligible men were randomized to receive finasteride 5 mg daily or placebo daily for a planned 7 years. Men were screened annually with a DRE and PSA. The PSA measurement for patients on finasteride was adjusted because of the effect of 5α-reductase inhibitors on the reading. If patients were found to have an abnormal DRE or an elevated PSA (4.0 ng/ml or higher), a prostate biopsy was recommended. Biopsy was performed transrectally using ultrasound guidance and a minimum of six cores was obtained. If the prostate biopsy was positive, men were removed from the study. If the biopsy was negative, they would continue on the protocol. All men who had not been diagnosed with prostate cancer at the end of the study (7 years) were offered a biopsy.

Follow-up: Median follow-up not reported; planned 7 years of treatment or until diagnosis of prostate cancer on biopsy

Endpoints: Prevalence of prostate cancer, biopsy recommendation rates, rates of nonadherence to treatment, and medication side effects

RESULTS:

- More than one-third of men randomized were 65 years of age or older (38.0%, n = 7,175).

- Of the 9,060 patients included in the final analysis, prostate cancer was diagnosed in 18.4% (n = 803) in the finasteride group and 24.4% (n = 1,147) in the placebo group.
  - The relative risk reduction of finasteride treatment on prostate cancer diagnosis was 24.8% (95% confidence interval [CI], 18.6 to 30.6).
- Of all the prostate cancers that were diagnosed, there was a higher proportion of high-grade cancers (Gleason score of at least 7) in the finasteride group compared to the placebo group (37.0% vs. 22.2%, p < 0.001).
  - Once a man was diagnosed with cancer, the relative risk of high-grade cancer with finasteride was 1.65 (95% CI, 1.44 to 1.93).
- The rate of biopsy recommendation of abnormal DRE and/or PSA was significantly higher in the placebo group (24.8% vs. 22.5%, p < 0.001).
- The rate of nonadherence to treatment in the finasteride group was 14.5%.
- Side effects related to sexual functioning or the endocrine system such as a reduced volume of ejaculate, erectile dysfunction, loss of libido, and gynecomastia were more common in men taking finasteride.
- Lower urinary tract symptoms and associated adverse effects were more common in the placebo group.

Criticisms and Limitations: The detection rate of prostate cancer was quite high; many of the per-protocol biopsy-detected cancers might not have become clinically significant during the patient's lifetime. The study did not address the more important oncological outcomes of disease-specific and overall survival.

Other Relevant Studies and Information:

- The REDUCE trial was a similar trial using dutasteride, which is also a phosphodiesterase-5 inhibitor (PDE-5). The study randomized men at high risk for prostate cancer (50 to 75 years of age, PSA 2.5 to 10.0 ng/ml, and one negative prostate biopsy) to receive either dutasteride or placebo for 4 years.[2] It found a similar relative risk reduction of 22.8% (95% CI, 15.2 to 29.8).
- In 2011, the US Food and Drug Administration (FDA) issued a safety warning about the possibly increased risk of high-grade prostate cancer related to the use of both PDE-5 inhibitors.[3]
- Secondary analyses of PCPT outcomes have indicated that long-term outcomes up to a median of 18.4 years favor the finasteride arm and suggest that the risk of high-risk cancer is not increased.[4,5]

- Linkage analysis of participants from PCPT to Medicare claims data also suggests no adverse long-term cardiac, endocrine, or sexual effects.[6]
- The SELECT trial evaluated the use of selenium and vitamin E to prevent prostate cancer and found that while selenium had no effect (hazard ratio [HR] 1.09, 95% CI, 0.93 to 1.27), vitamin E may actually increase the risk of developing prostate cancer (HR 1.17, 95% CI, 1.004 to 1.36).[7]

Summary and Implications: This study was the first to demonstrate an effective chemopreventive agent for prostate cancer with a large reduction in incidence with finasteride administration. However, the increased diagnosis of high-grade cancers triggered concern and curbed the enthusiasm for using finasteride for chemoprevention among urologists.

CLINICAL CASE: MANAGEMENT OF LOW-RISK PROSTATE CANCER

Case History:
A 60-year-old man with no family history of prostate cancer, a normal DRE, and a PSA of 2.1 ng/ml presents to the urologist seeking advice regarding lowering his risk of prostate cancer.

Suggested Answer:
This patient has a relatively low lifetime risk of developing prostate cancer, especially clinically significant disease. While findings from the PCPT trial as well as subsequent follow-up analyses would suggest that administering this patient finasteride would decrease his relative risk by nearly 25%, this does not represent a use approved by the FDA or the European Medicines Agency. Current guidelines from the European Association of Urology make a strong recommendation against the use of specific preventive or dietary measures for prostate cancer.[8]

References

1. Thompson IM, Goodman PJ, Tangen CM, et al. The influence of finasteride on the development of prostate cancer. *N Engl J Med.* 2003;349(3):215–24.
2. Andriole GL, Bostwick DG, Brawley OW, et al. Effect of dutasteride on the risk of prostate cancer. *N Engl J Med.* 2010;362(13):1192–202.
3. US Food and Drug Administration. FDA drug safety communication: 5-alpha reductase inhibitors (5-ARIs) may increase the risk of a more serious form of prostate

cancer. 2011; safety announcement. Available at: https://www.fda.gov/Drugs/DrugSafety/ucm258314.htm. Accessed 5/21/2019.

4. Goodman PJ, Tangen CM, Darke AK, et al. Long-term effects of finasteride on prostate cancer mortality. *N Engl J Med.* 2019;380(4):393–4.

5. Thompson IM, Jr., Goodman PJ, Tangen CM, et al. Long-term survival of participants in the Prostate Cancer Prevention Trial. *N Engl J Med.* 2013;369(7):603–10.

6. Unger JM, Hershman DL, Till C, et al. Using Medicare claims to examine long-term prostate cancer risk of finasteride in the Prostate Cancer Prevention Trial. *J Natl Cancer Inst.* 2018;110(11):1208–15.

7. Klein EA, Thompson IM, Jr., Tangen CM, et al. Vitamin E and the risk of prostate cancer: the Selenium and Vitamin E Cancer Prevention Trial (SELECT). *JAMA.* 2011;306(14):1549–56.

8. Mottet N, Bellmunt J, Bolla M, et al. EAU-ESTRO-SIOG guidelines on prostate cancer. Part 1: screening, diagnosis, and local treatment with curative intent. *Eur Urol.* 2017;71(4):618–29.

3

MRI-Targeted or Standard Biopsy for Prostate Cancer Diagnosis

The PRECISION Trial

PHILIPP DAHM

"The use of risk assessment with MRI before biopsy and MRI-targeted biopsy was superior to standard transrectal ultrasonography–guided biopsy [for identifying clinically significant prostate cancer] in men at clinical risk for prostate cancer who had not undergone biopsy previously."[1]

Research Question: In patients with a clinical suspicion of prostate cancer who have not undergo a prior biopsy, how does magnetic resonance imaging (MRI), with or without targeted biopsy, compare to standard transrectal ultrasound-guided (TRUS) biopsy in detecting clinically significant prostate cancer?

Funding: The National Institute for Health Research and the European Association of Urology Research Foundation

Year Study Began: February 2016

Year Study Published: 2018

Study Location: 25 centers in 11 countries

Who Was Studied: Men who had not undergone a prior biopsy with a clinical suspicion of prostate cancer based on an elevated prostate-specific antigen (PSA) level, an abnormal digital rectal examination (DRE), or both

Who Was Excluded: Men with a PSA of greater than 20 ng/ml, DRE findings concerning for extracapsular disease, or inability to undergo prostate biopsy or MRI

Patients: 500

Study Overview:

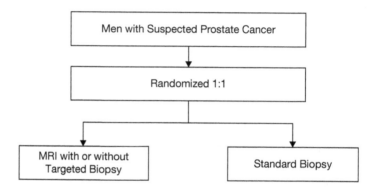

Study Interventions: Patients in the intervention arm underwent multiparametric MRI with the use of a 1.5T or 3.0T scanner with a pelvic phased-array coil, with or without an endorectal coil. Areas on the MRI scan suggestive of prostate cancer were categorized by a local radiologist according to the Prostate Imaging–Reporting and Data System, version 2 (PI-RADS v2), on a scale from 1 to 5, with higher numbers indicating a greater likelihood of clinically significant cancer. Men who had a positive result on the multiparametric MRI, namely an area scored 3 (equivocal regarding the likelihood of prostate cancer), 4 (likely to be prostate cancer), or 5 (highly likely to be prostate cancer), underwent MRI-targeted biopsy of up to three areas with up to four biopsies in each with the use of real-time ultrasonographic guidance. MRI biopsy target registration was performed by means of visual registration or software-assisted registration. Patients with lesions scored only 1 or 2 did not undergo biopsy. Patients in the control group underwent standard ultrasound-guided biopsy for a total of 10 to 12 biopsy cores.

Follow-up: Participants were followed until the visit at which their treatment decisions were made or until their 30-day postintervention questionnaires were completed, whichever was later.

Endpoints: Primary outcome: proportion of men with clinically significant prostate cancer, defined as the presence of a single biopsy core indicating disease of Gleason score 3 + 4 (Gleason sum of 7) or greater (Gleason sum of 8, 9, or 10). Secondary outcomes: proportion of men with clinically insignificant cancer (Gleason score 3 + 3), proportion of men in the MRI-targeted biopsy group who did not undergo biopsy, and proportion of men with adverse events after the intervention.

RESULTS:

- The mean patient age was approximately 64 years and the median PSA was 6.6 ng/ml.
- Clinically significant cancer was detected in 95 men (38%) in the MRI-targeted biopsy group and 64 (26%) in the standard biopsy group (absolute risk reduction 12.0; 95% confidence interval [CI], 4 to 20).
- A diagnosis of clinically insignificant cancer was made in 23 (9%) men versus 55 (22%) men in the MRI versus standard biopsy groups, respectively.
- A total of 2% of patients in either group experienced serious adverse events.
- Common patient-reported events such as blood in urine (30% vs. 63%) and rectal bleeding (14% vs. 22%) were less common in the MRI-targeted group, reflecting lower biopsy rates.

Criticism and Limitations: The trial was based on surrogate outcomes of prostate cancer pathology rather than disease-specific survival. While this trial was not limited to specialist centers, accurate MRI interpretation requires dedicated skills and training, and it is unclear how these findings translate into routine clinical practice.

Other Relevant Studies and Information:

- This study was preceded by the PROMIS study by the same investigators that evaluated the diagnostic accuracy of multiparametric MRI and TRUS biopsy in prostate cancer.[2] It found that multiparametric MRI was more sensitive (93%; 95% CI, 88 to 96) than TRUS biopsy (48%; 95% CI, 42 to 55) but less specific (41% [95% CI, 36 to 46] for multiparametric MRI vs. 96% [95% CI, 94 to 98] for TRUS biopsy). The authors suggested that multiparametric MRI be introduced as a triage test before first prostate biopsy to reduce unnecessary biopsies.

- An earlier study compared targeted MRI/ultrasound fusion biopsy with standard extended-sextant ultrasound-guided biopsy and found increased detection of high-risk prostate cancer and decreased detection of low-risk prostate cancer.[3]
- A study comparing MRI-directed targeted biopsy to systematic biopsy found that targeted biopsies may miss only 9% of unfavorable intermediate-risk or worse cancers.[4]
- Current evidence-based guidelines by the European Association of Urology now recommend multiparametric MRI in men with an elevated PSA prior to prostate biopsy.[5]

Summary and Implications: This study provided high-quality evidence to support the use of multiparametric MRI in men with an elevated PSA as a triage test to help determine the need for a biopsy. It has spurred widespread adoption of this imaging modality worldwide.

CLINICAL CASE: MULTIPARAMETRIC MRI IN MEN WITH AN ELEVATED PSA

Case History:
A 62-year-old Caucasian man with few health issues approached his primary care doctor about PSA screening. Understanding the risks and benefits and based on his personal circumstances, values, and preferences, he ultimately elected to undergo prostate cancer screening. His PSA is noted to be 7.8 ng/ml; after this value is confirmed by repeat testing 2 weeks later, he is referred to a urologist. His DRE reveals a prostate of about 35 g with no nodules. He has no family history of prostate cancer.

Suggested Answer:
Based on his PSA, the patient should undergo further diagnostic workup. Whereas a number of biomarkers have become available that may help better quantify his personal risk, the supporting evidence is not as convincing as that provided for multiparametric MRI.

In the absence of contraindications for undergoing MRI, this would be an excellent next step. Based on the results of the PROMIS study and assuming a pretest probability of 9% for harboring clinically significant prostate cancer, a negative multiparametric MRI would reduce his post-test probability to 2%. A positive MRI would increase his post-test probability to 14%, which is not that different. However, based on the PRECISION trial, an MRI-guided prostate biopsy is more likely to identify only those cancers that are clinically meaningful, thereby mitigating the issue of overdiagnosis and overtreatment.

References

1. Kasivisvanathan V, Rannikko AS, Borghi M, et al. MRI-targeted or standard biopsy for prostate-cancer diagnosis. *N Engl J Med* 2018;378(19):1767–77. doi: 10.1056/ NEJMoa1801993 [published online first: 2018/03/20]
2. Ahmed HU, El-Shater Bosaily A, Brown LC, et al. Diagnostic accuracy of multi-parametric MRI and TRUS biopsy in prostate cancer (PROMIS): a paired validating confirmatory study. *Lancet* 2017;389(10071):815–22. doi: 10.1016/S0140-6736(16)32401-1 [published online first: 2017/01/24]
3. Siddiqui MM, Rais-Bahrami S, Turkbey B, et al. Comparison of MR/ultrasound fusion-guided biopsy with ultrasound-guided biopsy for the diagnosis of prostate cancer. *JAMA* 2015;313(4):390–7. doi: 10.1001/jama.2014.17942 [published online first: 2015/01/28]
4. Ahdoot M, Wilbur AR, Reese SE, et al. MRI-targeted, systematic, and combined biopsy for prostate cancer diagnosis. *N Engl J Med* 2020;382(10):917–28. doi: 10.1056/NEJMoa1910038 [published online first: 2020/03/05]
5. Mottet N, van den Bergh RCN, Briers E, et al. Guidelines on prostate cancer 2020 [cited 2020 3/20/2020]. Available from: https://uroweb.org/guideline/prostate-cancer/.

4

Long-Term Survival Among Men With Conservatively Treated Localized Prostate Cancer

Conservative Management of Prostate Cancer

NIRANJAN SATHIANATHEN AND PHILIPP DAHM

"Men aged 65 to 75 years with conservatively treated low-grade prostate cancer incur no loss of life expectancy."[1]

Research Question: What is the risk of dying from prostate cancer of men with clinically localized prostate cancer managed conservatively with immediate or delayed hormone therapy?

Funding: Agency for Health Care Policy and Research, Rockville, MD, USA

Year Study Began: 1971

Year Study Published: 1995

Study Location: 37 acute hospitals and 2 Veterans Affairs medical centers in Connecticut

Who Was Studied: Men diagnosed with clinically localized prostate cancer who were aged 65 to 75 years at the time of diagnosis and were untreated or treated with immediate or delayed hormonal therapy

Who Was Excluded: Men with metastatic disease or obvious extracapsular extension, if there was no cancer on pathology re-review, diagnoses made at autopsy, diagnoses made incidentally at the time of bladder cancer treatment, and/ or if patients were treated with local curative therapy. Exclusions were also made if patient records could not be located, if pathology reports/slides were not available to confirm diagnoses, and/or if the treatment provided to a patient could not be determined.

Patients: 451

Study Overview:

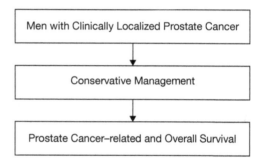

Study Interventions: In this observational study from the Connecticut Tumor Registry, men diagnosed with clinically localized prostate cancer from 1971 to 1976 who did not undergo curative treatment were followed up until time of death. The cause of death was obtained from death certificates.

Follow-up: Mean 15.5 years

Endpoint: Age-specific survival

RESULTS:

- After a mean 15.5 years of follow-up, 9% (n = 40) were alive, 34% (n = 154) had died of prostate cancer, and 49% (n = 221) had died of other causes.

- No men with low-grade disease (Gleason score 2 to 4) died within 7 years of diagnosis.
- Gleason score of tumor and comorbidity score were the first and second most powerful predictors of age-specific, all-cause mortality.
- Men with low-grade disease (Gleason score 2 to 4) treated conservatively had comparable survival outcomes to the general population.
- In patients with high-grade disease (Gleason score 8 to 10), 46% and 51% had died of prostate cancer within 10 and 15 years of diagnosis, respectively.

Criticisms and Limitations: This study predates the prostate-specific antigen (PSA) testing era and therefore mostly describes the outcomes of men with clinically detected prostate cancer or those incidentally diagnosed at the time of transurethral resection of the prostate (TURP) for benign prostatic hyperplasia. Today's patients are likely to experience more favorable outcomes due to lead time bias. Since that time there has been a major shift in the application of the Gleason grade scoring system, with Gleason scores of less than 6 no longer being used by pathologists; such reclassification may have led to an apparent improvement in outcomes over time.[2] As a single-armed study without a comparator, the results are unable to inform the question as to how these patients may have fared with other treatment modalities.

Other Relevant Studies and Information:

- Results of this study have since been updated to provide 20-year follow-up data.[3] It found that men with low Gleason grade cancers (Gleason score 2 to 4) had a 6 (95% confidence interval [CI], 2 to 11) per 1,000 risk of dying from prostate cancer over 20 years, which did not support aggressive treatment. In contrast, men with high-risk prostate cancer (Gleason score 8 to 10) had a 121 (95% CI, 90 to 156) per 1,000 risk of dying from prostate cancer.[3]
- The SPCG-4 study randomized men from the pre-PSA era to surgery or watchful waiting and thereby included a similar cohort of men. Whereas long-term follow-up of 29 years demonstrated a consistent oncological benefit of radical prostatectomy over watchful waiting, an exploratory subgroup analysis found age (less than 65 years vs. 65 years and older) to be an important effect modifier, with older patients experiencing a small benefit in disease-specific survival and less likely to experience an overall survival benefit.[4]

- The PIVOT trial from the early PSA era randomized men to surgery or watchful waiting and thereby also included a cohort of men who did not undergo local treatment with curative intent.[5] After nearly 20 years of follow-up there was only a small benefit in favor of radical prostatectomy group (absolute risk difference: 4% [95% CI, −0.2 to 8.3]; hazard ratio, 0.63 [95% CI, 0.39 to 1.02]; p = 0.06), which did not meet the predefined threshold of statistical significance.
- The results of this study have helped inform evidence-based guidelines by the American Urological Association and the European Association of Urology on the role of watchful waiting in men with a limited life expectancy.[6,7]

Summary and Implications: The findings from this study were important in establishing the safety of conservative management/watchful waiting for low-grade prostate cancer, especially in older men and/or those with comorbidities, by showing that their favorable survival outcomes with conservative management that was not very different from that of the general population. This supported the indolent nature of low-grade disease and the notion that subjecting these patients to curative therapy likely represented overtreatment.

CLINICAL CASE: MANAGEMENT OF LOW-GRADE PROSTATE CANCER IN ELDERLY MEN AND THOSE WITH COMORBIDITIES

Case History:
A 74-year-old man presents to the clinic seeking an opinion on management shortly after he was diagnosed with Gleason score 3 + 3, Gleason Grade Group 1 prostate cancer incidentally diagnosed at the time of TURP chips. The prostate cancer involves 15% of the TURP chips; his PSA is 3.4 ng/ml and his digital rectal exam is normal (clinical stage: cT1b, NoMO). His past medical history is significant for myocardial infarction requiring cardiac stent and type 2 diabetes mellitus with macro- and micro-vascular complications.

Suggested Answer:
This is an elderly man with multiple comorbidities and newly diagnosed, incidental, low-grade prostate cancer who, in accordance with current evidence-based guidelines, would be a suitable candidate for watchful waiting.[7,8]

Findings of a study by Albertsen et al.,[9] taken together with the results of the PIVOT trial,[5] would indicate that his risk of dying from prostate cancer is very low. At the same time, the patient can also be spared the side effects of local therapy. If employing a watchful waiting approach, patients should be appropriately counseled about the aims of this management option and should know that it is not curative.

References

1. Albertsen PC, Fryback DG, Storer BE, et al. Long-term survival among men with conservatively treated localized prostate cancer. *JAMA* 1995;274(8):626–31. doi: 10.1001/jama.1995.03530080042039

2. Albertsen PC, Hanley JA, Barrows GH, et al. Prostate cancer and the Will Rogers phenomenon. *J Natl Cancer Inst* 2005;97(17):1248–53. doi: 10.1093/jnci/dji248 [published online first: 2005/09/08]

3. Albertsen PC, Hanley JA, Fine J. 20-year outcomes following conservative management of clinically localized prostate cancer. *JAMA* 2005;293(17):2095–101. doi: 10.1001/jama.293.17.2095 [published online first: 2005/05/05]

4. Bill-Axelson A, Holmberg L, Garmo H, et al. Radical prostatectomy or watchful waiting in prostate cancer—29-year follow-up. *N Engl J Med* 2018;379(24):2319–29. doi: 10.1056/NEJMoa1807801 [published online first: 2018/12/24]

5. Wilt TJ, Jones KM, Barry MJ, et al. Follow-up of prostatectomy versus observation for early prostate cancer. *N Engl J Med* 2017;377(2):132–42. doi: 10.1056/NEJMoa1615869 [published online first: 2017/07/13]

6. Mottet N, Bellmunt J, Bolla M, et al. EAU-ESTRO-SIOG guidelines on prostate cancer. Part 1: screening, diagnosis, and local treatment with curative intent. *Eur Urol* 2017;71(4):618–29. doi: 10.1016/j.eururo.2016.08.003 [published online first: 2016/08/30]

7. Sanda MG, Cadeddu JA, Kirkby E, et al. Clinically localized prostate cancer: AUA/ASTRO/SUO guideline. Part II: recommended approaches and details of specific care options. *J Urol* 2018;199(4):990–97. doi: 10.1016/j.juro.2018.01.002 [published online first: 2018/01/15]

8. Cornford P, Bellmunt J, Bolla M, et al. EAU-ESTRO-SIOG guidelines on prostate cancer. Part II: treatment of relapsing, metastatic, and castration-resistant prostate cancer. *Eur Urol* 2017;71(4):630–42. doi: 10.1016/j.eururo.2016.08.002 [published online first: 2016/09/07]

9. Albertsen PC, Hanley JA, Gleason DF, et al. Competing risk analysis of men aged 55 to 74 years at diagnosis managed conservatively for clinically localized prostate cancer. *JAMA* 1998;280(11):975–80.

Clinical Results of Long-Term Follow-Up of a Large, Active Surveillance Cohort With Localized Prostate Cancer

NIRANJAN SATHIANATHEN

"We observed a low rate of prostate cancer mortality. Among the patients who were reclassified as higher risk and who were treated, PSA failure was relatively common. Other-cause mortality accounted for almost all of the deaths."[1]

Research Question: In patients with clinically localized, favorable-risk prostate cancer (Gleason score 6 or less, prostate-specific antigen [PSA] 10 ng/ml or less), what are the outcomes of active surveillance?

Funding: None reported

Year Study Began: November 1995

Year Study Published: January 2010

Study Location: Toronto, Canada

Who Was Studied: Men diagnosed with clinically localized, favorable-risk prostate cancer (Gleason score 6 or less, PSA 10 ng/ml or less). In the first 4 years of the study, men older than 70 years with a PSA up to 15 ng/ml or a Gleason score up to 3 + 4 were also included.

Who Was Excluded: Men with clinically advanced prostate cancer and/or those with intermediate- or high-risk disease

Patients: 450

Study Overview:

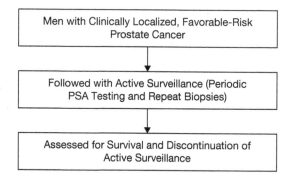

Study Interventions: This was a single-armed, prospectively planned cohort study.

- Men underwent PSA testing every 3 months for the first 2 years following diagnosis and then every 6 months thereafter.
- Patients also underwent an 8- to 14-core confirmatory biopsy at 6 to 12 months post-diagnosis and then every 3 to 4 years until they reached 80 years old.
- Disease reclassification was based on histological upgrade on repeat biopsy and/or clinical progression.
  - Histological upgrade was defined as the presence of Gleason score 7 disease or higher.
  - Clinical progression was defined as the development of a palpable nodule that was subsequently investigated with a biopsy and histological upgrade was confirmed.
  - A PSA doubling time less than 2 years was also used as a trigger for radical treatment during the first 4 years of the study, but the cutoff was changed to 3 years until 2009, from which it did not act as a trigger and instead was used as an indicator for further investigation with biopsy or multiparametric magnetic resonance imaging (MRI).

Follow-up: Median follow-up of 6.8 years

Endpoints: Overall survival, cause-specific survival, time to stopping active surveillance, time to PSA failure

---

RESULTS:

- The median age of patients was 70.3 years; 83% had Gleason score 6 disease or less.
- 97 of the 450 patients (21.6%) died during follow-up, all but three (0.6%) from causes other than prostate cancer.
- 135 patients (30.0%) stopped active surveillance. The main reasons were a short PSA doubling time (14.4%), Gleason grade progression (8.0%), and patient preference (4.0%).

Criticism and Limitations:

- As a single-arm study that assessed the prognosis of men with favorable-risk prostate cancer managed by active surveillance, the study lacked a comparison group. The study did not provide direct evidence as to how these patients may have fared had they undergone radical treatment or watchful waiting/observation without curative intent.
- Inclusion/exclusion criteria as well as the details of the active surveillance protocol changed several times during the study period. This includes revision of the Gleason grading system in 2005, which may have resulted in a proportion of Gleason score 6 patients being reclassified as higher grade.[2]

Other Relevant Studies and Information:

- The same authors reported an extension of this study for a cohort of 993 men and follow-up data up to 15 years that confirmed these findings.[3]
- Several other large international cohorts, including those that had different inclusion criteria and follow-up protocols, also reported satisfactory outcomes for active surveillance.[4–6]
- No trial comparing active surveillance to radical treatment exists; the Surveillance Therapy Against Radical Treatment (START) trial, which opened in 2007, was stopped early for failure to accrue.[7]

- The Prostate Cancer Intervention Versus Observation Trial (PIVOT) randomized men from the early PSA era to radical prostatectomy or watchful waiting and found only small, nonsignificant differences in survival outcomes after a median follow-up of 12 years, suggesting that many men undergoing active surveillance could be safely managed with watchful waiting.[8]
- The Prostate Testing for Cancer and Treatment (ProtecT) trial randomized screen-detected men with localized prostate cancer to active monitoring, radical prostatectomy, or radiotherapy.[9] After a mean follow-up of 10 years, there were few deaths from prostate cancer and outcomes of the three groups were similar.
- Evidence-based guidelines by the American Urological Association and the European Association of Urology now recommend active surveillance as the preferred approach for men with very-low-risk and low-risk prostate cancer.[10,11]

Summary and Implications: This study established the favorable outcomes of active surveillance as a management strategy for men with low-risk prostate cancer. As long as patients are carefully monitored, local treatment with curative intent can be safely deferred long term in many patients.

CLINICAL CASE: MANAGEMENT OF LOW-RISK PROSTATE CANCER WITH ACTIVE SURVEILLANCE

Case History:

A 65-year-old man with hypertension and no other significant medical or family history is diagnosed with Gleason $3 + 3 = 6$ (Grade Group 1) in 2 of 12 cores from a transurethral ultrasound-guided biopsy and has a PSA of 5.3 ng/ml.

Suggested Answer:

In accordance with current evidence-based guidelines, for a relatively young and otherwise healthy man with low-risk prostate cancer, active surveillance of his prostate cancer is recommended.[10,12] This and other studies have shown this to be a safe strategy in these patients, with a very low risk of cancer-specific mortality even with extended follow-up. These men are more likely to die from other causes than their low-risk cancer.

If conservative management is opted for, it is important that these men are followed up appropriately to assess for disease progression so that the window of curability is not missed. A confirmatory biopsy at 6 to 12 months is recommended for risk reassessment. In addition to regular PSA testing, magnetic resonance imaging and molecular biomarkers are being increasingly used to aid risk stratification and decision making. An upgrade in risk category should trigger reconsideration of local treatment with curative treatment.

References

1. Klotz L, Zhang L, Lam A, et al. Clinical results of long-term follow-up of a large, active surveillance cohort with localized prostate cancer. *J Clin Oncol* 2010;28(1):126–31. doi: 10.1200/JCO.2009.24.2180

2. Epstein JI, Allsbrook WC, Jr., Amin MB, et al. The 2005 International Society of Urological Pathology (ISUP) consensus conference on Gleason grading of prostatic carcinoma. *Am J Surg Pathol* 2005;29(9):1228–42. [published online first: 2005/08/13]

3. Klotz L, Vesprini D, Sethukavalan P, et al. Long-term follow-up of a large active surveillance cohort of patients with prostate cancer. *J Clin Oncol* 2015;33(3):272–7. doi: 10.1200/JCO.2014.55.1192

4. Tosoian JJ, Mamawala M, Epstein JI, et al. Intermediate and longer-term outcomes from a prospective active-surveillance program for favorable-risk prostate cancer. *J Clin Oncol* 2015;33(30):3379–85. doi: 10.1200/JCO.2015.62.5764 [published online first: 2015/09/02]

5. Welty CJ, Cowan JE, Nguyen H, et al. Extended follow-up and risk factors for disease reclassification in a large active surveillance cohort for localized prostate cancer. *J Urol* 2015;193(3):807–11. doi: 10.1016/j.juro.2014.09.094 [published online first: 2014/09/28]

6. Newcomb LF, Thompson IM, Jr., Boyer HD, et al. Outcomes of active surveillance for clinically localized prostate cancer in the prospective, multi-institutional Canary PASS cohort. *J Urol* 2016;195(2):313–20. doi: 10.1016/j.juro.2015.08.087 [published online first: 2015/09/04]

7. Klotz LH. Observation or radical treatment in patients with prostate cancer. ClinicalTrials.gov, 2007. https://clinicaltrials.gov/ct2/show/NCT00499174

8. Wilt TJ, Jones KM, Barry MJ, et al. Follow-up of prostatectomy versus observation for early prostate cancer. *N Engl J Med* 2017;377(2):132–42. doi: 10.1056/NEJMoa1615869 [published online first: 2017/07/13]

9. Hamdy FC, Donovan JL, Lane JA, et al. 10-year outcomes after monitoring, surgery, or radiotherapy for localized prostate cancer. *N Engl J Med* 2016;375(15):1415–24. doi: 10.1056/NEJMoa1606220 [published online first: 2016/09/15]

10. Mottet N, Bellmunt J, Bolla M, et al. EAU-ESTRO-SIOG guidelines on prostate cancer. Part 1: screening, diagnosis, and local treatment with curative intent. *Eur Urol* 2017;71(4):618–29. doi: 10.1016/j.eururo.2016.08.003 [published online first: 2016/08/30]

11. Sanda MG, Cadeddu JA, Kirkby E, et al. Clinically localized prostate cancer: AUA/ASTRO/SUO guideline. Part I: risk stratification, shared decision making, and care

options. *J Urol* 2018;199(3):683–90. doi: 10.1016/j.juro.2017.11.095 [published online first: 2017/12/06]

12. Sanda MG, Cadeddu JA, Kirkby E, et al. Clinically localized prostate cancer: AUA/ ASTRO/SUO guideline. Part II: recommended approaches and details of specific care options. *J Urol* 2018;199(4):990–97. doi: 10.1016/j.juro.2018.01.002 [published online first: 2018/01/15]

6

Radical Prostatectomy Versus Observation in Early Prostate Cancer

Scandinavian Prostate Cancer Group Study Number 4 (SPCG-4)

PHILIPP DAHM

"In this randomized trial [involving men with clinically localized prostate cancer], radical prostatectomy significantly reduced disease-specific mortality but there was no significant difference between surgery and watchful waiting in terms of overall survival."[1]

Research Question: In patients with clinically diagnosed prostate cancer from the era prior to prostate-specific antigen (PSA) testing, how does radical prostatectomy compare to watchful waiting?

Funding: Swedish Cancer Society

Year Study Began: October 1989

Year Study Published: September 2002

Study Location: 14 centers in Sweden, Finland, and Iceland

Who Was Studied: Men with clinically localized prostate cancer (stage T1-T2, N0M0) graded as well or moderately differentiated per the World Health

Organization classification of 1980. Men had to be less than 75 years of age with an estimated life expectancy of at least 10 years.

Who Was Excluded: Men with signs of metastases as documented on a bone scan or a urogram with signs of obstruction. Men with a PSA greater than 50 ng/ml were also excluded.

Patients: 698

Study Overview:

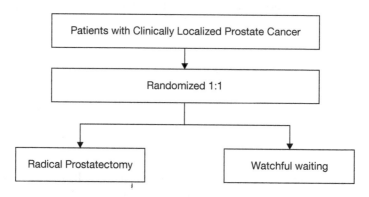

Study Interventions: Patients in the intervention arm underwent a pelvic lymph node dissection with frozen-section evaluation; only if the nodes were negative did patients undergo a retropubic prostatectomy. In the watchful waiting arm, patients underwent no immediate treatment.

Adjuvant local or systemic treatment was not given. Transurethral resection was recommended in the watchful waiting group for local progression. For men with local progression in the radical prostatectomy group, orchiectomy or treatment with gonadotropin-releasing hormones was recommended. Treatment for disseminated disease was the same in both groups. Follow-up included an annual PSA, bone scan, and chest radiograph.

Follow-up: Median follow-up of 6.2 years at the time of initial publication

Endpoints: Primary outcome: prostate cancer mortality. Secondary outcomes: metastases-free survival and risk of local tumor progression. Post hoc, death from any cause was added as an endpoint.

RESULTS:

- The mean patient age was approximately 65 years and the mean PSA was approximately 13 ng/ml; about 75% of men in each arm had clinically detectable (clinical stage T2) disease.
- In the surgery group, 26 of the 347 (4.7%) men died of prostate cancer; in the observation group, 31 of the 348 (8.9%) men died of prostate cancer.
- Death from any cause occurred in 53 (15.3%) and 62 (17.8%) men, respectively.

Table 6.1 Summary of the PIVOT Key Findings

Outcome	Surgery	Observation	Hazard Ratio (95% CI)	Absolute Risk Reduction (95% CI) at 8 Years
Death from prostate cancer	4.6%	8.9%	0.50 (0.27 to 0.91)	6.6% (2.1 to 11.1)
Death from any cause	15.3%	17.8%	0.83 (0.57 to 1.2)	6.3% (−0.2 to 12.7)
Local progression	11.5%	31.0%	0.31 (0.22 to 0.44)	41.8% (35.2 to 48.4)
Distant metastases	10.1%	15.5%	0.63 (0.41 to 0.96)	13.9% (8.0 to 19.8)

Data from reference 2.

Criticism and Limitations: A majority of men enrolled in this trial from the pre-PSA era had palpable disease by digital rectal examination (DRE). This differs from today's patients, who mostly have PSA-detected disease, thereby limiting the generalizability of findings. The definition of local progression in the watchful waiting group included "symptoms of obstruction of the flow of urine that necessitated intervention"; benign prostatic hyperplasia may have contributed to the high event rate in this group.

Other Relevant Studies and Information:

- A companion paper reported on quality-of-life findings from this trial and found that urinary incontinence and erectile dysfunction were more common and urinary obstruction was less common in the radical prostatectomy group.[3]

- Extended follow-up to a median follow-up of 23.6 years has since been reported. The risk ratio for dying from prostate cancer was 0.55 (95% confidence interval [CI], 0.41 to 0.74), corresponding to an absolute risk reduction (ARR) of 11.7% (95% CI, 5.2 to 18.2). The risk of all-cause mortality was also substantially reduced; risk ratio: 0.74 (95% CI, 0.62 to 0.87); ARR: 12.0% (95% CI, 5.5 to 18.4).[4]
- The Prostate Cancer Intervention Versus Observation Trial (PIVOT) was similar as it randomized men from the early PSA era to radical prostatectomy versus observation (Table 6.1). After a median follow-up of 12.7 years, there was a small, nonsignificant difference in favor of surgery (hazard ratio, 0.63; 95% CI, 0.39 to 1.02); ARR: 4.0% (95% CI, –0.2 to 8.3).[2]
- The Prostate Testing for Cancer and Treatment (ProtecT) trial compared radical prostatectomy to radiation therapy and active monitoring.[5,6] At 10 years of follow-up, this study failed to show a benefit of surgery.
- Evidence-based guidelines by the American Urological Association and the European Association of Urology recommend radical prostatectomy as a suitable treatment choice for men with low-risk prostate cancer unwilling to undergo active surveillance, those with favorable and unfavorable intermediate-risk prostate cancer, and those with high-risk prostate cancer.[7,8]

Summary and Implications: This study provides the central evidentiary support for recommending radical prostatectomy as treatment in patients with clinically localized prostate cancer. Its findings are best generalized to patients with clinically detectable disease with an extended life expectancy of 15 years or greater. These findings may not be directly applicable anymore, however, because this study was initiated in the pre-PSA era and involved men with palpable disease by DRE.

CLINICAL CASE: RADICAL PROSTATECTOMY VERSUS OBSERVATION IN CLINICALLY LOCALIZED PROSTATE CANCER

Case History:

A 59-year-old patient without significant medical comorbidity undergoes a screening DRE notable for a prominent one-sided nodule. His PSA is found to be 18 ng/ml. He is found to have Gleason score 4 + 4 (Grade Group 4)

prostate cancer in a total of 8 of 12 cores bilaterally. A staging computed tomographic scan and bone scan are negative for evidence of metastatic disease.

Suggested Answer:

This patient's presentation is notable for several factors that portend a poor
long-term risk, most notably his Gleason score, DRE findings, his PSA level,
and his prostate cancer volume. Given his relative youth, good health, and lack
of medical comorbidities, he should undergo local treatment with curative intent. SPCG-4 provides evidence to support a long-term benefit of surgery over
watchful waiting, particularly in younger patients. Surgery also leaves open the
option of adjuvant or salvage radiation at a later time if his disease recurs.

References

1. Holmberg L, Bill-Axelson A, Helgesen F, et al. A randomized trial comparing radical prostatectomy with watchful waiting in early prostate cancer. *N Engl J Med*
   2002;347(11):781–9. doi: 10.1056/NEJMoa012794 [published online first: 2002/
   09/13]
2. Wilt TJ, Jones KM, Barry MJ, et al. Follow-up of prostatectomy versus observation for Early Prostate Cancer. *N Engl J Med* 2017;377(2):132–42. doi: 10.1056/
   NEJMoa1615869 [published online first: 2017/07/13]
3. Steineck G, Helgesen F, Adolfsson J, et al. Quality of life after radical prostatectomy or
   watchful waiting. *N Engl J Med* 2002;347(11):790–6. doi: 10.1056/NEJMoa021483
   [published online first: 2002/09/13]
4. Bill-Axelson A, Holmberg L, Garmo H, et al. Radical prostatectomy or watchful
   waiting in prostate cancer—29-year follow-up. *N Engl J Med* 2018;379(24):2319–
   29. doi: 10.1056/NEJMoa1807801 [published online first: 2018/12/24]
5. Donovan JL, Hamdy FC, Lane JA, et al. Patient-reported outcomes after monitoring,
   surgery, or radiotherapy for prostate cancer. *N Engl J Med* 2016;375(15):1425–37.
   doi: 10.1056/NEJMoa1606221 [published online first: 2016/09/15]
6. Hamdy FC, Donovan JL, Lane JA, et al. 10-Year Outcomes after Monitoring, Surgery,
   or Radiotherapy for Localized Prostate Cancer. *N Engl J Med* 2016;375(15):1415–
   24. doi: 10.1056/NEJMoa1606220 [published online first: 2016/09/15]
7. Mottet N, Bellmunt J, Bolla M, et al. EAU-ESTRO-SIOG Guidelines on Prostate
   Cancer. Part 1: Screening, Diagnosis, and Local Treatment with Curative Intent.
   Eur Urol 2017;71(4):618–29. doi: 10.1016/j.eururo.2016.08.003 [published online
   first: 2016/08/30]
8. Sanda MG, Cadeddu JA, Kirkby E, et al. Clinically Localized Prostate Cancer: AUA/
   ASTRO/SUO Guideline. Part I: Risk Stratification, Shared Decision Making,
   and Care Options. *J Urol* 2018;199(3):683–90. doi: 10.1016/j.juro.2017.11.095
   [published online first: 2017/12/06]

7

Radical Prostatectomy Versus Observation for Localized Prostate Cancer

The Prostate Cancer Intervention Versus Observation Trial (PIVOT)

PHILIPP DAHM

"Among men with localized prostate cancer detected during the early era of PSA testing, radical prostatectomy did not significantly reduce all-cause or prostate-cancer mortality, as compared with observation, through at least 12 years of follow-up."[1,2]

Research Question: In patients with a diagnosis of clinically localized prostate cancer from the early prostate-specific antigen (PSA) testing era, how does radical prostatectomy compare to observation?

Funding: Department of Veterans Affairs Cooperative Studies Program (and others)

Year Study Began: November 1994

Year Study Published: July 2012

Study Location: 44 Department of Veterans Affairs sites and 8 National Cancer Institute sites in the United States

Who Was Studied: Men with clinically localized prostate cancer (stage T1-T2, NxM0 of any grade). Men had to be medically fit for radical prostatectomy, be aged 75 years or less, and have an estimated life expectancy of at least 10 years.

Who Was Excluded: Men with a PSA of 50 ng/ml or greater or suggestion of metastatic disease based on a bone scan

Patients: 731

Study Overview:

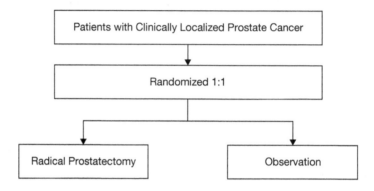

Study Interventions: Patients in the intervention arm underwent radical prostatectomy using an approach at the surgeon's discretion, most commonly radical retropubic prostatectomy. Additional interventions (such as radiation therapy or hormonal therapy) was also determined at each participant's and his physician's discretion. Men in the observation arm did not receive any specific treatment. They were offered palliative hormonal or chemotherapy for symptomatic or metastatic disease at their provider's discretion.

Follow-up: Median follow-up of 10.0 years for initial publication[1] and 12.7 years for follow-up publication[2]

Endpoints: Primary outcome: all-cause mortality. Secondary outcomes: prostate cancer mortality (defined as death definitely or probably due to prostate cancer or treatment based on assessment by a masked adjudication committee); local, regional, or systemic progression; urinary incontinence, erectile dysfunction, and bowel dysfunction of at least moderate severity.

RESULTS:

- Mean patient age was 67 years and median PSA was 7.8 ng/ml.
- In the surgery group, 223 of the 364 (61.3%) men died; in the observation group, 245 of the 367 (66.8%) men died (Table 7.1).
- Death attributed to prostate cancer or treatment occurred in 27 men (7.4%) assigned to the surgery arm and 42 men (11.4%) assigned to observation.
- In the surgery group, 149 men (40.9%) experienced local, regional, or systemic disease progression. In the observation group, 251 men (68.4%) progressed.
- In the surgery group, 53 (14.6%) and 63 men (17.3%) experienced erectile dysfunction and urinary incontinence, respectively. In the observation group, the corresponding figures were 20 (5.4%) and 16 (4.4%), respectively.
- A 20-year follow-up analysis of PIVOT found that "surgery was not associated with significantly lower all-cause or prostate-cancer mortality than observation [but surgery] was associated with a higher frequency of adverse events." At the 20-year mark, the surgical group did have "a lower frequency of treatment for disease progression, mostly for asymptomatic, local, or biochemical progression."

Table 7.1 SUMMARY OF THE PIVOT KEY FINDINGS

Outcome	Surgery	Observation	Hazard Ratio (95% Confidence Interval)	Absolute Risk Reduction (95% Confidence Interval)
Death from any cause	61.3%	66.8%	0.92 (0.82 to 1.02)	5.5% (−1.5 to 12.4)
Death from prostate cancer	7.4%	11.4%	0.65 (0.42 to 1.03)	4.0% (−0.2 to 8.3)
Any disease progression	40.9%	68.4%	0.39 (0.32 to 0.48)	27.5% (20.4 to 34.2)
Treatment for any disease progression	33.5%	59.7%	0.45 (0.36 to 0.56)	26.2% (19.0 to 32.9)
Erectile dysfunction	14.6%	5.4%	2.77 (1.65 to 4.63)	−9.1% (−13.5 to −4.8)
Urinary incontinence	17.3%	4.4%	4.22 (2.44 to 7.3)	−12.9 (−17.5 to −8.6)

Data from reference 2.

Criticism and Limitations: The trial was underpowered, as reflected in the wide confidence intervals for most outcomes, in particular for the subgroup analyses performed. It also dates back to the early PSA era and included men with fairly high PSA values with potentially undetected (micro-) metastatic disease.

Other Relevant Studies and Information:

- Longer-term follow-up (median follow-up of survivors: 18.6 years) for overall survival has since been reported.[3] The updated study found that surgery may also provide small reductions in death from any cause and increases in years of life gained. Based on subgroup analyses, absolute effects were small in men with low-risk disease, greater in men with intermediate-risk disease, and not apparent in men with high-risk disease
- The other important trial informing the comparison of radical prostatectomy to observation is the Scandinavian Prostate Cancer Group Trial 4 (SPCG-4),[4] which dates back to the pre-PSA era. This study indicated a substantial benefit of surgery over observation with long-term follow-up.
- The Prostate Testing for Cancer and Treatment (ProtecT) trial compared radical prostatectomy to radiation therapy and active monitoring.[5,6] At 10 years of follow-up, this study failed to show a benefit of surgery.
- Based on these data, current evidence-based guidelines by the American Urological Association and the European Association of Urology emphasize shared decision making with an important role of active surveillance in men with low-risk and favorable intermediate-risk prostate cancer who are at low risk for disease-related morbidity and mortality.[7,8]

Summary and Implications: This study has drawn into question the widespread use of radical prostatectomy for clinically localized prostate cancer, especially in men with competing medical comorbidities and lower-risk disease. Patients with similar baseline characteristics as those enrolled in PIVOT are unlikely to achieve a substantial benefit at a median follow-up of up to 20 years but may experience substantial side effects.

CLINICAL CASE: RADICAL PROSTATECTOMY VERSUS OBSERVATION IN CLINICALLY LOCALIZED PROSTATE CANCER

Case History:

A 69-year-old patient with diabetes mellitus and coronary artery status post stent placement is found to have cT1N0M0 Gleason score 3 + 4 prostate cancer in 3 of 12 cores with up to 35% core involvement. His PSA is 7.5 ng/ml.

Suggested Answer:

PIVOT showed that there may be no benefit of surgery over observation in terms of overall mortality and disease-specific mortality. For many men, the risk of dying of something other than prostate cancer–related causes far exceeds their risk of dying from prostate cancer. A subset of patients may experience a small benefit in absolute terms; these men are likely those who have few competing comorbidities, have an extended life expectancy of at least 15 years, and have higher-risk disease.

Based on life expectancy calculators, the patient described in this case has a 45% risk of dying of other causes by 10 years of follow-up. He is unlikely to realize a survival benefit with regard to this risk of dying from prostate cancer with surgery but may also experience urinary incontinence and erectile dysfunction as a consequence. Therefore, surgery should not be recommended for this patient.

References

1. Wilt TJ, Brawer MK, Jones KM, et al. Radical prostatectomy versus observation for localized prostate cancer. *N Engl J Med* 2012;367(3):203–13. doi: 10.1056/NEJMoa1113162
2. Wilt TJ, Jones KM, Barry MJ, et al. Follow-up of prostatectomy versus observation for early prostate cancer. *N Engl J Med* 2017;377(2):132–42. doi: 10.1056/NEJMoa1615869 [published online first: 2017/07/13]
3. Wilt TJ, Vo TN, Langsetmo L, et al. Radical prostatectomy or observation for clinically localized prostate cancer: extended follow-up of the Prostate Cancer Intervention Versus Observation Trial (PIVOT). *Eur Urol* 2020 doi: 10.1016/j.eururo.2020.02.009 [published online first: 2020/02/25]
4. Bill-Axelson A, Holmberg L, Ruutu M, et al. Radical prostatectomy versus watchful waiting in early prostate cancer. *N Engl J Med* 2005;352(19):1977–84. doi: 10.1056/NEJMoa043739

5. Donovan JL, Hamdy FC, Lane JA, et al. Patient-reported outcomes after monitoring, surgery, or radiotherapy for prostate cancer. *N Engl J Med* 2016;375(15):1425–37. doi: 10.1056/NEJMoa1606221 [published online first: 2016/09/15]

6. Hamdy FC, Donovan JL, Lane JA, et al. 10-year outcomes after monitoring, surgery, or radiotherapy for localized prostate cancer. *N Engl J Med* 2016;375(15):1415–24. doi: 10.1056/NEJMoa1606220 [published online first: 2016/09/15]

7. Mottet N, Bellmunt J, Bolla M, et al. EAU-ESTRO-SIOG guidelines on prostate cancer. Part 1: screening, diagnosis, and local treatment with curative intent. *Eur Urol* 2017;71(4):618–29. doi: 10.1016/j.eururo.2016.08.003 [published online first: 2016/08/30]

8. Sanda MG, Cadeddu JA, Kirkby E, et al. Clinically localized prostate cancer: AUA/ASTRO/SUO guideline. Part I: risk stratification, shared decision making, and care options. *J Urol* 2018;199(3):683–90. doi: 10.1016/j.juro.2017.11.095 [published online first: 2017/12/06]

8

10-Year Outcomes After Monitoring, Surgery, or Radiotherapy

The Prostate Testing for Cancer and Treatment (ProtecT) Trial

PHILIPP DAHM

"At a median of 10 years, prostate-cancer-specific mortality was low irrespective of the treatment assigned, with no significant difference among treatments."[1]

Research Question: In patients with a diagnosis of clinically localized prostate cancer diagnosed by prostate-specific antigen (PSA) screening, how does radical prostatectomy compare to radiotherapy and active monitoring?

Funding: National Institute for Health Research in the United Kingdom

Year Study Began: 1999

Year Study Published: October 2016

Study Location: Eight academic hospitals in the United Kingdom

Who Was Studied: Men with clinically localized prostate cancer 50 to 69 years of age with an estimated life expectancy of 10 years

Who Was Excluded: Men with concomitant or past malignancy

Patients: 545

Study Overview:

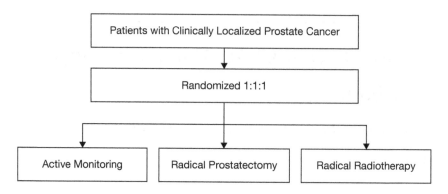

Study Interventions: Patients in the active monitoring arm deferred initial local treatment and were monitored clinically with PSA measurements every 3 months in the first year and every 6 to 12 months thereafter. A PSA increase of 50% or more over a 12-month period triggered review for consideration of continued monitoring, additional testing, radical treatment (surgery or radiation), or palliative management.

Radiotherapy included neoadjuvant androgen-deprivation therapy for 3 to 6 months before and concomitantly with three-dimensional conformal radiotherapy delivered at a total of 74 Gy in 37 fractions. A PSA rise by at least 2 ng/ml above the nadir was considered evidence of progression.

Follow-up: Median follow-up of 10.0 years

Endpoints: Primary outcome: prostate-cancer-related mortality, with prostate-cancer-related deaths defined as deaths that were definitely or probably due to prostate cancer or its treatment based on ascertainment by a blinded committee. Secondary outcomes: all-cause-mortality, rates of mortality, clinical progression, primary treatment failure, and treatment complications. Metastatic disease was defined as bony, visceral, or lymph node metastases on imaging or a PSA above 100 ng/ml. Treatment failure after surgery was defined as a PSA of 0.2 ng/ml at least 3 months after surgery, and treatment failure after radiotherapy was defined according to the Phoenix Consensus Conference recommendations as a rise by 2 ng/ml or more above the nadir.

RESULTS:

- Median age (range) was 62 (50 to 69) years.[2]
- 88% of the men assigned to active monitoring, 71% of the men assigned to surgery, and 74% of the men assigned to radiotherapy actually received the assigned treatment with 9 months after randomization.
- Of the men initially managed by active monitoring, 54.8% received radical treatment (surgery or radiation) by the end of follow-up.
- Few men in any of the three treatment arms died of prostate cancer: 8 (1.5%) in the active monitoring arm, 5 (0.9%) in the surgery arm, and 4 (0.7%) in the radiotherapy arm.
- The number of men who developed metastatic disease was 33 (6.0%), 13 (2.3%), and 16 (2.9%), respectively.
- The number of men who died of any cause was 59 (10.8%), 55 (9.9%), and 55 (10.1%), respectively.
- There were few serious complications in any treatment arm, in particular no death in the surgery arm.

Criticism and Limitations:

- Follow-up of this trial was relatively short at a median of 10 years, especially considering the low number of events. Differences between the treatment modalities may become apparent with longer follow-up.
- Active monitoring based largely on PSA follow-up is no longer used. Current active surveillance regimens rely on a combination of PSA monitoring, repeat prostate biopsies at certain intervals, and, increasingly, dedicated magnetic resonance imaging.[3]

Other Relevant Studies and Information:

- The Cluster Randomized Trial of PSA Testing (CAP) was an extension of the ProtecT trial that randomized primary care centers to either population-based PSA screening or standard United Kingdom National Health Service management without routine PSA testing. The trial did not demonstrate a benefit of one-time PSA screening at 10 years of follow-up.[4]
- Baseline characteristics of patients of the ProtecT trial are reported in a separate publication.[2]

- An accompanying publication reported the patient-reported outcomes such as urinary continence, erectile dysfunction, and quality of life from this trial.[5]
- Based on these data, current evidence-based guidelines by the American Urological Association and the European Association of Urology are emphasizing shared decision making with patients, with a greater role for active surveillance in those with low-risk and favorable intermediate-risk prostate cancer who are at low risk for disease-related morbidity and mortality.[6,7]

Summary and Implications: This study underscores the very low risk of death from prostate cancer irrespective of treatment approach in patients diagnosed by PSA screening. Radical surgery and radiation therapy should be reserved for men with higher-risk disease and an extended life expectancy of well beyond 10 years.

CLINICAL CASE: 10-YEAR OUTCOMES AFTER MONITORING, SURGERY, OR RADIOTHERAPY

Case History:

A 65-year-old patient with atrial fibrillation on apixaban is found to have cT1N0M0 Gleason score 3 + 4 prostate cancer in 2 of 12 cores with up to 10% core involvement. His PSA is 6.3 ng/ml. He is exploring treatment options that offer him the chance of long-term cure.

Suggested Answer:

The ProtecT trial demonstrated a very low risk of death from prostate cancer after a median of 10 years of follow-up. The patient has favorable intermediate-risk disease with low cancer volume. Given that he does not want to consider a watchful waiting approach, active surveillance as the contemporary version of active monitoring would be the preferred initial approach. While incurring the burden of frequent PSA testing, repeat biopsies, and magnetic resonance imaging, it avoids the side effects of radical surgery or radiation therapy.

References

1. Hamdy FC, Donovan JL, Lane JA, et al. 10-year outcomes after monitoring, surgery, or radiotherapy for localized prostate cancer. *N Engl J Med.* 2016; 375(15): 1415–24. doi:10.1056/NEJMoa1606220

2. Lane JA, Donovan JL, Davis M, et al. Active monitoring, radical prostatectomy, or radiotherapy for localised prostate cancer: Study design and diagnostic and baseline results of the ProtecT randomised phase 3 trial. *Lancet Oncol.* 2014; 15(10): 1109–18. doi:10.1016/S1470-2045(14)70361-4

3. Klotz L, Vesprini D, Sethukavalan P, et al. Long-term follow-up of a large active surveillance cohort of patients with prostate cancer. *J Clin Oncol.* 2015; 33(3): 272–277. doi:10.1200/JCO.2014.55.1192

4. Martin RM, Donovan JL, Turner EL, et al. Effect of a low-intensity PSA-based screening intervention on prostate cancer mortality: The CAP randomized clinical trial. *JAMA.* 2018; 319(9): 883–95. doi:10.1001/jama.2018.0154

5. Donovan JL, Hamdy FC, Lane JA, et al. Patient-reported outcomes after monitoring, surgery, or radiotherapy for prostate cancer. *N Engl J Med.* 2016; 375(15): 1425–37. doi:10.1056/NEJMoa1606221

6. Mottet N, Bellmunt J, Bolla M, et al. EAU-ESTRO-SIOG guidelines on prostate cancer. Part 1: Screening, diagnosis, and local treatment with curative intent. *Eur Urol.* 2017; 71(4): 618–29. doi:10.1016/j.eururo.2016.08.003

7. Sanda MG, Cadeddu JA, Kirkby E, et al. Clinically localized prostate cancer: AUA/ASTRO/SUO guideline. Part I: Risk stratification, shared decision making, and care options. *J Urol.* 2018; 199(3): 683–90. doi:10.1016/j.juro.2017.11.095

9

Comparative Effectiveness of Minimally Invasive Versus Open Radical Prostatectomy

PHILIPP DAHM

"Men undergoing minimally invasive radical prostatectomy vs. radical retropubic prostatectomy experienced shorter length of stay, fewer respiratory and miscellaneous surgical complications and strictures, and similar postoperative use of additional cancer therapies but experienced more genitourinary complications, incontinence, and erectile dysfunction."[1]

Research Question: In patients with clinically localized prostate cancer, how does minimally invasive prostatectomy compare to open retropubic prostatectomy?

Funding: Department of Defense Prostate Cancer Physician Training Award

Year Study Began: US Surveillance, Epidemiology, and End Results (SEER) Medicare-linked data from 2003 through 2007

Year Study Published: October 2009

Study Location: Population-based state registries contributing to SEER program

Who Was Studied: Men aged 65 years or older who were diagnosed as having prostate cancer from 2002 to 2005 and followed through December 2007

Who Was Excluded: Men not enrolled in a health maintenance organization or who were not enrolled in both Medicare Part A and Part B for the duration of the study (because claims were not reliably submitted for those patients). Also, men with prior other cancer diagnoses and those who underwent radical perineal prostatectomy.

Patients: 8,837

Study Overview:

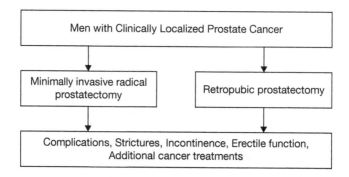

Study Interventions: Patients in the intervention arm underwent minimally invasive radical prostatectomy (MIRP) as identified by the *Current Procedural Terminology,* Fourth Edition (CPT-4), code 55866. Men in the control group underwent radical retropubic prostatectomy (RRP) as identified by codes 55840, 55842, and 55845. Propensity model adjustment was performed for year of surgery, age, comorbidity, baseline urinary incontinence, baseline erectile dysfunction, race/ethnicity, marital status, education, income, SEER region, population density, pathologic grade, and stage.

Follow-up: Median follow-up was 2.8 years (range: 1 day to 5 years).

Endpoints: Outcomes included length of stay, transfusions, 30-day complications, anastomotic strictures, incontinence, erectile function, additional prostate cancer treatment, and mortality.

RESULTS:

- The study included 1,938 MIRP patients and 6,899 RRP patients; the proportion of MIRP rose from 9.2% in 2003 to 43.2% in 2006.

- Patients undergoing MIRP were more likely to have organ-confined disease (68.3% vs. 60.8%).
- In a propensity score–adjusted model, outcomes of both approaches were similar with several exceptions (Table 9.1):
  - Reported rates of a diagnosis of urinary incontinence (1.3; 95% confidence interval [CI], 1.05 to 1.72) and diagnosis of erectile dysfunction (1.4; 95% CI, 1.14 to 1.72) were higher in the MIRP group, but treatment rates for both issues were not statistically different.
  - Reported rates of anastomotic strictures (0.38; 95% CI, 0.28 to 0.52) and blood transfusions (0.11; 95% CI, 0.06 to 0.17) were lower for MIRP, and length of stay was also shorter (0.67 days; 95% CI, 0.58 to 0.72).
- The study did not report outcomes for prostate cancer–specific survival.

Table 9.1 PROPENSITY MODEL–ADJUSTED OUTCOMES BY SURGICAL APPROACH

Outcome	MIRP	RRP	Risk Ratio
Death*	0.8	0.9	0.91 (0.53–1.57)
Additional prostate cancer treatment*	8.2	6.9	1.19 (0.84–1.69)
Overall	5.1	4.9	1.05 (0.84–1.32)
Radiation	5.3	3.7	1.42 (0.88–2.32)
Hormone			
Incontinence*	15.9	12.2	1.3 (1.05–1.72)
Diagnosis	7.8	8.9	0.87 (0.69–1.1)
Treatment			
Erectile dysfunction*	26.8	19.2	1.40 (1.14–1.72)
Diagnosis	2.3	2.2	1.05 (0.74–1.51)
Treatment			
Anastomotic stricture (%)	5.8	14.0	0.38 (0.28–0.52)
30-day complications	22.3	23.2	0.95 (0.77–1.16)
Blood transfusion	2.7	20.8	0.11 (0.06–0.17)
Length of stay, median (IQR)	2(1–2)	3(2–4)	0.67 (0.58–0.72)

*During study period (per 100 person-years)

Criticism and Limitations:

- Since this was a retrospective observational study with short-term follow-up based on administrative data, it is possible that confounding factors influenced the results. Despite the use of a propensity model to adjust for confounders, residual confounding may have persisted.

- The authors were unable to distinguish between patients undergoing robotic-assisted laparoscopic surgery (RALP) versus "pure" laparoscopic surgery, although the contribution of the latter group was likely small.
- The study reflects the early community learning curve with the robotic approach by a generation of surgeons with limited procedure-specific experience.

Other Relevant Studies and Information:

- A study based on the Nationwide Inpatient Sample database found that the adoption of MIRP during the 2003–2006 timeframe of rapid adoption of the robotic approach found that patients undergoing MIRP in 2005 were more likely to encounter issues and complications (odds ratio: 2.0; 95% CI, 1.1 to 3.7) than those undergoing RRP as assessed by Agency for Healthcare Research and Quality Patient Safety Indicators.[2]
- Short-term perioperative[3] and patient-reported outcomes[4] of the first randomized trial have only been recently reported but did not address the outcome prostate cancer-specific survival. Based on this study, RALP likely results in little to no difference in urinary quality of life, sexual quality of life, and overall surgical complications.[5] It likely reduces length of stay and risk of transfusion.[5]
- To date, current evidence-based guidelines by the American Urological Association and the European Association of Urology do not favor one surgical approach over another.[6–8]

Summary and Implications: In the absence of randomized controlled trials comparing MIRP to RRP,[9] this study was the first high-quality observational study that sought to adjust for baseline confounding and compare the historical RRP approach to RALP. It found mixed results that favored MIRP in terms of some perioperative complications, rates of transfusions and length of stay, but favored the traditional RRP approach in terms of functional outcomes. Since this study was published, RALP has nevertheless become the de facto standard of care in the United States.

CLINICAL CASE: ROBOTIC-ASSISTED LAPAROSCOPIC VERSUS OPEN RETROPUBIC PROSTATECTOMY

Case History:

A 68-year-old patient with newly diagnosed cT1N0M0 Gleason score 4 + 3 (5 of 12 cores bilaterally; PSA 10.2 ng/ml) prostate cancer elects to undergo radical prostatectomy. He has no significant past medical history except for diet-controlled diabetes and hypertension for which he takes a single agent. His body mass index is 35 and he has had no prior abdominal surgery except for a right inguinal hernia repair with mesh. He has comprehensive healthcare insurance and lives in a metropolitan area where he has access to both open and robotic surgeons. Which approach should he choose?

Suggested Answer:

Neither American Urological Association[10] nor European Association of Urology[6] guidelines recommend a specific surgical approach. In contrast to the time when Hu et al.[1] published this study, robotic-assisted surgery teaching has been firmly integrated into both urology residency and fellowship training programs in the United States to an extent that recent graduates likely have higher proficiency and better skills in performing RALP than RRP. Whereas superior oncological and functional outcomes of contemporary RALP remain unproven, patients can expect a shorter length of stay and a reduced risk of transfusion than with RRP. Assuming he finds a skilled and experienced surgeon, the recommendation should be for this patient to undergo RALP.

References

1. Hu JC, Gu X, Lipsitz SR, et al. Comparative effectiveness of minimally invasive vs open radical prostatectomy. *JAMA* 2009;302(14):1557–64. doi: 10.1001/jama.2009.1451
2. Parsons JK, Messer K, Palazzi K, et al. Diffusion of surgical innovations, patient safety, and minimally invasive radical prostatectomy. *JAMA Surg* 2014;149(8):845–51. doi: 10.1001/jamasurg.2014.31 [published online first: 2014/07/06]
3. Yaxley JW, Coughlin GD, Chambers SK, et al. Robot-assisted laparoscopic prostatectomy versus open radical retropubic prostatectomy: early outcomes from a randomised controlled phase 3 study. *Lancet* 2016;388(10049):1057–66. doi: 10.1016/S0140-6736(16)30592-X [published online first: 2016/07/31]
4. Coughlin GD, Yaxley JW, Chambers SK, et al. Robot-assisted laparoscopic prostatectomy versus open radical retropubic prostatectomy: 24-month outcomes from a randomised controlled study. *Lancet Oncol* 2018;19(8):1051–60. doi: 10.1016/S1470-2045(18)30357-7 [published online first: 2018/07/19]

5. Ilic D, Evans SM, Allan CA, et al. Laparoscopic and robotic-assisted versus open radical prostatectomy for the treatment of localised prostate cancer. *Cochrane Database Syst Rev* 2017;9:CD009625. doi: 10.1002/14651858.CD009625.pub2 [published online first: 2017/09/13]

6. Mottet N, Bellmunt J, Bolla M, et al. EAU-ESTRO-SIOG guidelines on prostate cancer. Part 1: screening, diagnosis, and local treatment with curative intent. *Eur Urol* 2017;71(4):618–29. doi: 10.1016/j.eururo.2016.08.003 [published online first: 2016/08/30]

7. Mottet N, van den Bergh RCN, Briers E, et al. Guidelines on prostate cancer 2020 [cited 3/20/2020]. Available from: https://uroweb.org/guideline/prostate-cancer/
.

8. Sanda MG, Cadeddu JA, Kirkby E, et al. Clinically localized prostate cancer: AUA/ASTRO/SUO guideline. Part I: risk stratification, shared decision making, and care options. *J Urol* 2018;199(3):683–90. doi: 10.1016/j.juro.2017.11.095 [published online first: 2017/12/06]

9. Kang DC, Hardee MJ, Fesperman SF, et al. Low quality of evidence for robot-assisted laparoscopic prostatectomy: results of a systematic review of the published literature. *Eur Urol* 2010;57(6):930–7. doi: 10.1016/j.eururo.2010.01.034 [published online first: 2010/02/09]

10. Sanda MG, Cadeddu JA, Kirkby E, et al. Clinically localized prostate cancer: AUA/ASTRO/SUO guideline. Part II: recommended approaches and details of specific care options. *J Urol* 2018;199(4):990–97. doi: 10.1016/j.juro.2018.01.002 [published online first: 2018/01/15]

10

Quality of Life and Satisfaction With Outcome Among Prostate Cancer Survivors

Quality of Life After Primary Treatment of Localized Prostate Cancer

NIRANJAN SATHIANATHEN AND PHILIPP DAHM

"Each prostate-cancer treatment was associated with a distinct pattern of change in quality-of-life domains related to urinary, sexual, bowel, and hormonal function."[1]

Research Question: What are the quality-of-life outcomes of men with clinically localized prostate cancer undergoing radical prostatectomy, brachytherapy, or external-beam radiotherapy as primary treatment?

Funding: National Institutes of Health

Year Study Began: 2003

Year Study Published: 2008

Study Location: Nine university-affiliated hospitals in the United States

Who Was Studied: Men with prostate cancer who had chosen to undergo prostatectomy, brachytherapy, or external-beam radiotherapy as primary treatment. Partners of these men were also studied.

Who Was Excluded: Men who had received any treatment for their prostate cancer prior to prostatectomy, brachytherapy, or external-beam radiotherapy

Patients: 1,201 patients and 625 spouses or partners

Study Overview:

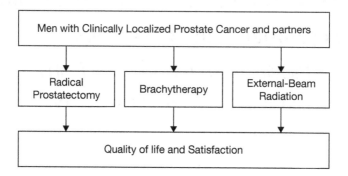

Study Interventions: This prospective, nonrandomized cohort study compared three groups of men with localized prostate cancer who elected to undergo radical prostatectomy, brachytherapy, or external-beam radiotherapy. These men were administered the Expanded Prostate Cancer Index Composite (EPIC-26) and Service Satisfaction Scale for Cancer Care (SCA) at defined timepoints after 2, 6, 12, and 24 months. Partners of men included were also studied through the Service Satisfaction Scale for Cancer Care for Partners (SCA-P) and EPIC–Partner tools, which were administered at 2, 6, 12, and 24 months.

Follow-up: Median 30 months

Endpoints: Quality-of-life domains at defined time intervals over time, baseline factors that affected changes in quality of life within study groups, impact of changes in quality of life on partner distress, relative effect of various domain changes of quality of life on overall outcome

---

RESULTS:

- The study enrolled 603 radical prostatectomy, 292 external-beam radiotherapy, and 306 brachytherapy patients. It also included 625 partners (99% of them female).

- Patients differed in baseline characteristics. Surgery patients were on average younger, had less comorbid disease, and had less severe prostate cancer.
- Each treatment modality had its own unique profile in terms of functional and quality-of-life outcomes (Table 10.1):
  - Urinary incontinence and sexual function were worst in surgery patients in the short term but subsequently improved; the extent of nerve sparing influenced recovery of sexual function and to some extent urinary continence.
  - Sexual functional outcomes were poorest in patients who were older and had a large prostate and/or a high pretreatment prostate-specific antigen (PSA) score.
  - Both urinary irritation scores and bowel function were negatively affected by both external-beam therapy and brachytherapy in the short term but subsequently improved.

Table 10.1 PERCENTAGE OF PATIENTS AND THEIR PARTNERS REPORTING A "BIG PROBLEM" OR "MODERATE PROBLEM" RELATED TO CERTAIN SYMPTOM DOMAINS AT 1 YEAR FOLLOWING TREATMENT

	Radical Prostatectomy		Brachytherapy		External-Beam Radiotherapy	
	Patient	Partner	Patient	Partner	Patient	Partner
Sexual function	26%	21%	16%	6%	16%	10%
Urinary incontinence	8%	5%	5%	5%	4%	3%
Urinary irritation or obstruction	12%	3%	18%	7%	14%	3%
Bowel or rectal function	2%	<2%	10%	4%	11%	5%
Vitality or hormone function	9%	15%	25%	17%	18%	15%

Criticisms and Limitations: The lack of randomization (as also reflected in the substantial difference in baseline characteristics) limits direct comparability across the three groups. The overall response rate at 2 years was only 61%, thereby introducing potential attrition bias. Participants of this study were recruited from tertiary care centers, and all three treatment approaches have since evolved further; both issues limit the generalizability of this study's results to today's patients.

Other Relevant Studies and Information:

- The Prostate Cancer Outcomes Study (PCOS) study is a population-based study of men with localized prostate cancer between the ages of 55 and 74 years who had undergone either surgery (1,164 men) or radiotherapy (491 men).[2] Patients undergoing prostatectomy were more likely to have urinary incontinence than were those undergoing radiotherapy at 5 years (odds ratio, 5.10; 95% confidence interval [CI], 2.29 to 11.36) and to experience sexual dysfunction at 5 years (odds ratio, 1.96; 95% CI, 1.05 to 3.63). Surgical patients were less likely to have bowel urgency.
- The Prostate Testing for Cancer and Treatment (ProtecT) trial randomized men with localized cancer to either active monitoring, surgery, or radiotherapy.[3] There were no large differences between the groups in quality of life. Urinary incontinence was worst in surgery patients. Voiding symptoms were worse in the radiotherapy group at 6 months but then recovered to be similar to baseline and other groups. Erectile function decreased in all groups but was worst in the prostatectomy group compared to other treatments. Bowel function and bother scores were not affected in the surgery or active monitoring group but were worse in the radiotherapy group.
- Supported by data from this study, current evidence-based guidelines by the American Urological Association (AUA) and the European Association of Urology strongly emphasize shared decision making when it comes to treatment.[4,5]

Summary and Implications: This study defined the unique impact of prostatectomy, external-beam radiotherapy, and brachytherapy on quality-of-life domains related to urinary, sexual, bowel, and hormonal function. Importantly, patient quality of life had an impact on partner satisfaction.

CLINICAL CASE: IMPACT OF PRIMARY PROSTATE CANCER TREATMENT ON QUALITY OF LIFE

Case History:

A 60-year-old man with localized Gleason 4 + 3, Gleason Grade Group 3, prostate adenocarcinoma in very good overall health is being counseled about his treatment options and the impact of each on his quality of life. He is already aware of the oncological efficacy of each management option. He is otherwise well and is sexually active. He does have considerable lower urinary tract symptoms, with an AUA symptom score of 17 (on a scale of 0 to 25, with a higher score indicating worse symptoms).

Suggested Answer:

This study provides detailed insights into the unique side-effect and quality-of-life profiles of three major treatment modalities that are valuable for patient counseling. The patient's treatment choice will very much depend on his individual values and preferences. One factor that speaks in favor of surgery are his preexisting urinary tract symptoms, likely due to benign prostatic hyperplasia, which would likely be alleviated by surgery and worsened by radiation. Downsides of surgery are the risk of both transient and longer-term urinary incontinence. A reduction in erectile function could be mitigated by a nerve-sparing approach. Ultimately, the patient needs to be assisted in making a treatment decision that is consistent with his own priorities.

References

1. Sanda MG, Dunn RL, Michalski J, et al. Quality of life and satisfaction with outcome among prostate-cancer survivors. *N Engl J Med* 2008;358(12):1250–61. doi: 10.1056/NEJMoa074311

2. Resnick MJ, Koyama T, Fan KH, et al. Long-term functional outcomes after treatment for localized prostate cancer. *N Engl J Med* 2013;368(5):436–45. doi: 10.1056/NEJMoa1209978 [published online first: 2013/02/01]

3. Donovan JL, Hamdy FC, Lane JA, et al. Patient-reported outcomes after monitoring, surgery, or radiotherapy for prostate cancer. *N Engl J Med* 2016;375(15):1425–37. doi: 10.1056/NEJMoa1606221 [published online first: 2016/09/15]

4. Mottet N, Bellmunt J, Bolla M, et al. EAU-ESTRO-SIOG guidelines on prostate cancer. Part 1: screening, diagnosis, and local treatment with curative intent. *Eur Urol* 2017;71(4):618–29. doi: 10.1016/j.eururo.2016.08.003 [published online first: 2016/08/30]

5. Sanda MG, Cadeddu JA, Kirkby E, et al. Clinically localized prostate cancer: AUA/ASTRO/SUO guideline. Part I: risk stratification, shared decision making, and care options. *J Urol* 2018;199(3):683–90. doi: 10.1016/j.juro.2017.11.095 [published online first: 2017/12/06]

11

Adjuvant Radiotherapy for Pathologically Advanced Prostate Cancer

A Southwest Oncology Group Randomized Controlled Trial (SWOG 8794)

PHILIPP DAHM

"In men who had undergone radical prostatectomy for pathologically advanced prostate cancer, adjuvant radiotherapy resulted in significantly reduced risk of PSA relapse and disease recurrence, although the improvements in metastasis-free survival and overall survival were not statistically significant."[1]

Research Question: In patients with pT3N0M0 prostate cancer, does adjuvant radiotherapy improve metastasis-free survival?

Funding: National Cancer Institutes of the United States and Canada

Year Study Began: August 1988

Year Study Published: November 2006

Study Location: Multiple institutions in the United States and Canada (not further described)

Who Was Studied: Men who had undergone radical prostatectomy within 16 weeks prior to randomization with a negative bone scan but one or more criteria for extra-prostatic disease:

- Extracapsular tumor extension
- Positive surgical margins
- Seminal vesicle invasion

Patients were required to have a pelvic lymph node dissection (except those at very low risk). An undetectable prostate-specific antigen (PSA) level was not required at the time of enrollment.

Who Was Excluded: Men with involvement of the pelvic lymph nodes and those with surgical complications such as total urinary incontinence, rectal injury, urinary extravasation, or pelvic infection.

Patients: 425

Study Overview:

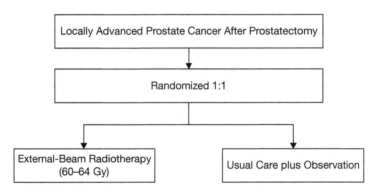

Study Interventions: Patients in the intervention arm underwent external-beam radiotherapy to the pelvic fossa at a dose of 60 to 64 Gy in 30 to 32 fractions within 10 working days after randomization. Patients in the control arm were followed expectantly.

Follow-up: Median follow-up of 10.6 years

Endpoints: Primary outcome: metastasis-free survival, defined as time to first occurrence of metastatic disease or death due to any cause. Secondary outcomes: PSA relapse, recurrence-free survival, overall survival, freedom from hormonal therapy, and postoperative complications.

RESULTS:

- 67% of patients had extracapsular extension or positive margins; 10% had seminal vesicle invasion.
- Approximately half the patients (of 302 with available data) had a PSA of 10 ng/ml or more prior to surgery.
- Only a subset of patients (249/425; 56.6%) had a documented undetectable PSA of 0.2 ng/ml or less after prostatectomy prior to radiation; in 49 patients the PSA status prior to adjuvant radiation therapy was unknown.
- 76 of the 214 (35.5%) patients in the adjuvant radiotherapy group and 91 of the 211 (43.1%) patients in the observation group developed metastases or died (hazard ratio [HR] 0.75; 95% confidence interval [CI], 0.55 to 1.02) (Table 11.1). This corresponded to median survival times of 14.7 years versus 13.2 years, respectively.
- Rates of biochemical progression (defined as PSA of more than 0.4 ng/ml) were reported in 60 of the 172 (34.9%) patients in the adjuvant radiotherapy group versus 112 of the 175 (64.0%) patients in the observation group (HR 0.43; 95% CI, 0.31 to 0.58).
- Recurrence-free survival also favored the adjuvant radiotherapy group; overall survival was not significantly different.
- Complications were more common in the radiotherapy group (23.8% vs. 11.9%; risk ratio 2.0; 95% CI, 1.3 to 3.1). Complications included proctitis or rectal bleeding, urethral strictures, and total urinary incontinence.

Table 11.1 SUMMARY OF THE SWOG 8794 TRIAL

Outcome	Adjuvant Radiotherapy	Observation	Hazard Ratio (95% CI)
Metastasis-free survival	35.5%	43.1%	0.75 (0.55 to 1.02)
Biochemical progression (PSA > 0.4 ng/ml)*	34.9%	64.0%	0.43 (0.31 to 0.58)
Recurrence-free survival	39.3%	52.6%	0.62 (0.46 to 0.82)
Overall survival	33.2%	39.3%	0.80 (0.58 to 1.09)

*Limited to 376 patients with PSA data available

Criticism and Limitations: In over 40% of patients the PSA level was either detectable or unknown prior to adjuvant radiotherapy; therefore, a considerable proportion of patients actually received salvage radiotherapy rather than adjuvant radiotherapy. There was substantial crossover: 16 patients in the radiotherapy group either did not receive any radiation or received less than the intended dose, and 70 men in the observation group received radiotherapy at some point. The number of metastatic events was substantially lower than anticipated, thereby limiting the statistical power of the analyses.

Other Relevant Studies and Information:

- Extended follow-up to a median of 12.6 years has since been reported, demonstrating significant differences favoring adjuvant radiotherapy for both metastasis-free survival (HR 0.71; 95% CI, 0.54 to 0.94) and overall survival (0.72; 95% CI, 0.55 to 0.96).[2]
- Two other trials have addressed the question of adjuvant radiotherapy: European Organisation for Research and Treatment of Cancer (EORTC) 22911[3] and the German ARO 96-02,[4] which was the only trial in which all patients had an undetectable PSA at the time of adjuvant radiotherapy. Neither study demonstrated a positive impact on metastasis-free survival or overall survival, although biochemical recurrence-free survival was improved.
- Preliminary results of the Radiation Therapy and Androgen Deprivation Therapy in Treating Patients Who Have Undergone Surgery for Prostate Cancer (RADICALS-RT) trial,[5] which included a comparison of adjuvant radiation therapy versus salvage radiation therapy, suggest that early salvage radiotherapy is preferred.
- Collaborative guidelines by the American Society of Radiation Oncology and the American Urological Association state that physicians should offer adjuvant radiotherapy to patients with adverse pathologic findings at prostatectomy including seminal vesicle invasion, positive surgical margins, or extra-prostatic extension.[6]

Summary and Implications: SWOG 8794 is the main study suggesting a benefit of adjuvant radiotherapy among patients with prostate cancer and adverse pathologic findings including seminal vesicle invasion, positive surgical margins, and extra-prostatic extension.[6][7] The tradeoffs of adjuvant radiotherapy are the acute and late genitourinary and gastrointestinal toxicity of radiotherapy and the potential overtreatment of patients who may never experience biochemical recurrence or complications from recurrent prostate cancer.

CLINICAL CASE: ADJUVANT RADIOTHERAPY

Case History:

A 54-year-old patient with no chronic illnesses undergoes robotic-assisted laparoscopic prostatectomy for cT1N0M0 Gleason score 3 + 4 (Grade Group 3) prostate cancer in 3 of 12 cores bilaterally. His prostatectomy pathology demonstrates pT3aN0, indicating extracapsular extension. Margins are focally positive at the right base and apex. Both an initial postprostatectomy PSA at 4 weeks and a follow-up value at 3 months are undetectable. While he continues to have erectile dysfunction, his continence is much improved, requiring only one or two pads daily. He is referred to radiation oncology for consideration of adjuvant radiotherapy.

Suggested Answer:

Extracapsular extension and positive margins are both adverse pathologic features that increase the patient's risk of biochemical recurrence and, ultimately, the development of locally recurrent disease as well as distant lymph node and bone metastases. An alternative approach to adjuvant radiotherapy would be close follow-up and prompt salvage radiotherapy in the setting of biochemical recurrence. However, to date, no published trial evidence is available to compare salvage radiotherapy to observation or, more importantly, adjuvant versus salvage radiotherapy. Given the patient's pathologic features and extended life expectancy, adjuvant radiotherapy should be considered, recognizing an increased risk of radiation-related side effects and impaired urinary and sexual quality of life both in the long term and the short term.

References

1. Thompson IM, Jr., Tangen CM, Paradelo J, et al. Adjuvant radiotherapy for pathologically advanced prostate cancer: a randomized clinical trial. *JAMA* 2006;296(19):2329–35. doi: 10.1001/jama.296.19.2329
2. Thompson IM, Tangen CM, Paradelo J, et al. Adjuvant radiotherapy for pathological T3N0M0 prostate cancer significantly reduces risk of metastases and improves survival: long-term followup of a randomized clinical trial. *J Urol* 2009;181(3):956–62. doi: 10.1016/j.juro.2008.11.032 [published online first: 2009/01/27]
3. Bolla M, van Poppel H, Tombal B, et al. Postoperative radiotherapy after radical prostatectomy for high-risk prostate cancer: long-term results of a randomised controlled trial (EORTC trial 22911). *Lancet* 2012;380(9858):2018–27. doi: 10.1016/S0140-6736(12)61253-7 [published online first: 2012/10/23]
4. Wiegel T, Bottke D, Steiner U, et al. Phase III postoperative adjuvant radiotherapy after radical prostatectomy compared with radical prostatectomy alone in pT3 prostate

cancer with postoperative undetectable prostate-specific antigen: ARO 96-02/AUO AP 09/95. *J Clin Oncol* 2009;27(18):2924–30. doi: 10.1200/JCO.2008.18.9563 [published online first: 2009/05/13]

5. Radiation Therapy and Androgen Deprivation Therapy in Treating Patients Who Have Undergone Surgery for Prostate Cancer (RADICALS). ClinicalTrials.gov, 2020. Available from: https://clinicaltrials.gov/ct2/show/NCT00541047, accessed 3/20/2020.

6. Thompson IM, Valicenti RK, Albertsen P, et al. Adjuvant and salvage radio-therapy after prostatectomy: AUA/ASTRO Guideline. *J Urol* 2013;190(2):441–9. doi: 10.1016/j.juro.2013.05.032 [published online first: 2013/05/28]

7. Cornford P, Bellmunt J, Bolla M, et al. EAU-ESTRO-SIOG guidelines on prostate cancer. Part II: treatment of relapsing, metastatic, and castration-resistant prostate cancer. *Eur Urol* 2017;71(4):630–42. doi: 10.1016/j.eururo.2016.08.002 [published online first: 2016/09/07]

12

Survival Following Primary Androgen Deprivation Therapy Among Men With Localized Prostate Cancer

JOSEPH ZABELL

"Primary androgen deprivation is not associated with improved survival among the majority of elderly men with T1-T2 prostate cancer."[1]

Research Question: In patients with a diagnosis of clinically localized prostate cancer, how does primary androgen deprivation therapy (ADT) improve disease-specific survival and overall survival?

Funding: National Cancer Institute

Year Study Began: 1992

Year Study Published: 2008

Study Location: Data derived from Surveillance, Epidemiology, and End Results (SEER) Medicare-linked database

Who Was Studied: Patients over the age of 66 who were diagnosed with T1-T2 prostate cancer between 1992 and 2002 and who did not receive local therapy (prostatectomy or radiation) within 180 days of initial diagnosis

Who Was Excluded: Patients without both Medicare Part A (hospitalization) and Part B (physician and outpatient) as their primary healthcare insurance coverage during the study period. Also excluded were patients with missing data, unknown cancer grade, or initiation of ADT before cancer diagnosis.

Patients: 19,271

Study Overview:

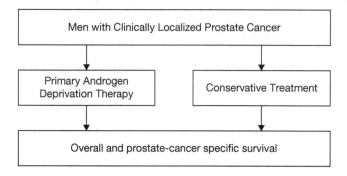

Study Interventions: This was a population-based study comparing men who received primary ADT (intervention of interest) or were treated conservatively. The investigators using instrumental variable analysis based on health service areas as a sophisticated statistical approach to account for potential confounding. Multivariable analysis was performed including the variables age, race, comorbidity status, cancer stage, cancer grade, income status, urban residence, marital status, and year of diagnosis.

Follow-up: Median follow-up was 81 months

Endpoints: Primary outcome: overall and prostate-cancer specific survival

RESULTS:

- The median patient age was 79 years in the primary ADT group and 77 in the conservative management group.
- The primary ADT group had a greater proportion of patients with poorly differentiated (34.2% vs. 14.2%) and T2 disease (50.2% vs. 35.8%).
- Based on instrumental variable analysis (IVA), primary ADT was associated with increased prostate cancer–specific mortality (hazard ratio

1.17; 95% confidence interval, 1.03 to 1.33). There was no significant effect on median overall survival (82 months vs. 82 months).

- Patients with poorly differentiated cancer demonstrated modestly improved prostate cancer–specific survival with primary ADT, but there was no effect on median overall survival.
- Based on a Cox multivariable model, prostate cancer–specific survival was also worse for patients treated with primary ADT compared to conservative treatment.
- Longer use of primary ADT was associated with lower prostate cancer–specific and overall survival in the subset of men treated for at least 3 years.

Criticism and Limitations: This was a retrospective observational study based on an administrative database that used advanced statistical methods to attempt to adjust statistically for both measured and unmeasured confounders and thereby mimic a randomized controlled trial; residual confounding is nevertheless likely to exist. In addition, the study only included patients 66 years of age or older and the median patient age was in the high 70s; thus, the results may not generalize to younger patients.

Other Relevant Studies and Information:

- A prior retrospective observational study based on the Cancer of the Prostate Strategic Urologic Endeavor (CaPSURE) national disease registry of men with prostate cancer suggested favorable disease control in patients receiving primary ADT. However, these findings were based on a small subset of patients and the study was unlikely to have adjusted for confounding variables.[2]
- During the 1990s, the use of primary ADT increased considerably among men who were 80 years of age or older and had low-risk, localized tumors.[3,4] A study attributed this non–evidence-based approach to the lucrative Medicare reimbursement policies for the administration of GNRH analogs.[5] The rate of inappropriate use of ADT declined after reimbursement was substantially reduced with the Medicare Modernization Act.
- Early ADT in conjunction with definitive radiotherapy has demonstrated a survival benefit for patients with high-risk prostate cancer.[6]

- Immediate hormone therapy for patients found to have positive lymph nodes at the time of prostatectomy has demonstrated improved survival in previous randomized trials.[7]

Summary and Implications: This study found no improvement in survival for men receiving primary ADT. While survival benefits of ADT have been identified in the setting of concurrent radiation therapy, node-positive disease, and metastatic prostate cancer, benefits in the primary setting are less clear. Furthermore, serious adverse impacts on quality of life[8] and cardiovascular complications[9] have been associated with ADT. Therefore, primary ADT is not recommended by major guidelines for the treatment of localized prostate cancer.[10]

CLINICAL CASE: PRIMARY ADT IN CLINICALLY LOCALIZED PROSTATE CANCER

Case History:

A 77-year-old male presents with newly diagnosed Gleason 4 + 3 prostate cancer with a prostate-specific antigen level of 12. Given his age and medical comorbidities, with an estimated life expectancy of less than 10 years, local treatment in the form of surgery and radiation does not appear indicated. Is there a role for primary ADT in this patient?

Suggested Answer:

This study would indicate no benefit to primary ADT in this patient with clinically localized prostate cancer who is unlikely to harbor metastatic disease. The outcomes of the watchful waiting arm of the Prostate Cancer Intervention Versus Observation Trial (PIVOT)[11] and long-term observational studies[12] would suggest a favorable outcome with observation alone.

References

1. Lu-Yao GL, Albertsen PC, Moore DF, et al. Survival following primary androgen deprivation therapy among men with localized prostate cancer. *JAMA*. 2008;300(2):173–181.
2. Kawakami J, Cowan JE, Elkin EP, et al. Androgen-deprivation therapy as primary treatment for localized prostate cancer: data from Cancer of the Prostate Strategic Urologic Research Endeavor (CaPSURE). *Cancer*. 2006;106(8):1708–1714.
3. Shahinian VB, Kuo YF, Freeman JL, et al. Increasing use of gonadotropin-releasing hormone agonists for the treatment of localized prostate carcinoma. *Cancer*. 2005;103(8):1615–1624.

4. Weight CJ, Klein EA, Jones JS. Androgen deprivation falls as orchiectomy rates rise after changes in reimbursement in the U.S. Medicare population. *Cancer*. 2008;112(10):2195–2201.

5. Shahinian VB, Kuo YF, Gilbert SM. Reimbursement policy and androgen-deprivation therapy for prostate cancer. *N Engl J Med*. 2010;363(19):1822–1832.

6. Bolla M, Collette L, Blank L, et al. Long-term results with immediate androgen suppression and external irradiation in patients with locally advanced prostate cancer (an EORTC study): a phase III randomised trial. *Lancet*. 2002;360(9327):103–106.

7. Messing EM, Manola J, Sarosdy M, et al. Immediate hormonal therapy compared with observation after radical prostatectomy and pelvic lymphadenectomy in men with node-positive prostate cancer. *N Engl J Med*. 1999;341(24):1781–1788.

8. Potosky AL, Reeve BB, Clegg LX, et al. Quality of life following localized prostate cancer treated initially with androgen deprivation therapy or no therapy. *J Natl Cancer Inst*. 2002;94(6):430–437.

9. Keating NL, O'Malley AJ, Smith MR. Diabetes and cardiovascular disease during androgen deprivation therapy for prostate cancer. *J Clin Oncol*. 2006;24(27):4448–4456.

10. Mottet N, Bellmunt J, Bolla M, et al. EAU-ESTRO-SIOG guidelines on prostate cancer. Part 1: screening, diagnosis, and local treatment with curative intent. *Eur Urol*. 2017;71(4):618–629.

11. Wilt TJ, Jones KM, Barry MJ, et al. Follow-up of prostatectomy versus observation for early prostate cancer. *N Engl J Med*. 2017;377(2):132–142.

12. Albertsen PC, Hanley JA, Fine J. 20-year outcomes following conservative management of clinically localized prostate cancer. *JAMA*. 2005;293(17):2095–2101.

Bilateral Orchiectomy With or Without Flutamide for Metastatic Prostate Cancer

PHILIPP DAHM

"The addition of flutamide to bilateral orchiectomy does not result in a clinically meaningful improvement in survival among patients with metastatic prostate cancer."[1]

Research Question: In patients with metastatic prostate cancer, how does addition of the anti-androgen flutamide to bilateral orchiectomy affect survival?

Funding: US National Cancer Institute and Southwest Oncology Group (SWOG)

Year Study Began: 1989

Year Study Published: 1998

Study Location: SWOG centers in the United States

Who Was Studied: Patients with histologically confirmed adenocarcinoma of the prostate with bone or distant soft tissue metastases, SWOG performance status of 0 to 3, and adequate renal function

Who Was Excluded: Patients who had undergone prior hormonal therapy, chemotherapy, or biological response modifiers

Patients: 1,387

Study Overview:

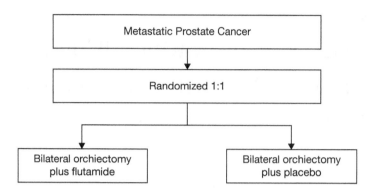

Study Interventions: Patients in the intervention arm received flutamide (125 mg given orally three times a day) in addition to bilateral orchiectomy; patient in the control group received placebo in addition to bilateral orchiectomy.

Patients underwent baseline history and physical as well as laboratory studies; these were repeated at months 1 and 3 and every 3 months thereafter. Computed tomography (CT) and bone scan were completed every 6 months for the first 2 years, and if the prostate-specific antigen (PSA) level rose above 25 ng/ml thereafter.

No guidelines for treatment after progression were provided, and crossover from placebo to flutamide was optional.

Follow-up: Median follow-up of 49.2 months (placebo group) and 50.1 months (flutamide group)

Endpoints: Primary outcome: overall survival. Secondary outcomes: progression-free survival and PSA response.

RESULTS:

- The mean patient age was 70 years in both groups. Median PSA was 130 and 193 ng/ml in the placebo and control group, respectively.
- Median overall survival was 29.9 months in the placebo group and 33.5 months in the flutamide group (hazard ratio [HR], 0.91; 95% confidence interval, 0.81 to 1.01; p = 0.14).

- Median progression-free survival was 18.6 months in the placebo group versus 20.4 months in the flutamide group (p = 0.26; no HR provided).
- There was also no significant difference in overall or progression-free survival between the flutamide and placebo groups in analyses stratified by disease extent.
- 43 patients (33 in the flutamide group and 10 in the placebo group) withdrew due to toxicity. The rate of grade 2 diarrhea was higher in the flutamide group (6.3% vs. 2.7%, p = 0.002). Rates of grade 2 anemia were 8.5% in the flutamide group and 5.4% in the placebo group (p = 0.024).

Criticism and Limitations: Compliance with flutamide in the intervention group and crossover in the control group were not assessed. Differences in subsequent treatment upon progression of disease were not accounted for and may have impacted outcomes. The wide confidence interval for overall survival, which is consistent with a potential benefit, indicates the study was underpowered.

Other Relevant Studies and Information:

- Findings of this trial conflicted with those of a prior trial that randomized 603 men with metastatic prostate cancer who were also randomized to flutamide versus placebo but received medical (rather than surgical) castration with leuprolide.[2] The flutamide group was favored both for median length of survival (35.6 vs. 28.3 months; p = 0.035) and median progression-free survival (16.5 vs. 13.9 months; p = 0.039).
- Individual patient meta-analyses of multiple randomized controlled trials that included the two anti-androgens nilutamide and flutamide indicated only a small benefit in favor of maximum androgen blockade at 5 years (27.6% vs. 24.7%; absolute risk difference 2.9%).

Summary and Implications: This study suggests no survival benefit but increased side effects from the addition of an anti-androgen such as flutamide to surgical castration among men with metastatic prostate cancer. While subsequent analyses[3] have suggested a small benefit of maximum androgen blockade using nonsteroidal anti-androgens, the benefit likely does not counterbalance the increased rate of adverse events.[4] In practice, anti-androgens are often used on a short-term basis at the time of initiation of treatment with luteinizing hormone–releasing hormone (LHRH) agonists to prevent symptom flare (from testosterone surge) in untreated patients with extensive metastatic disease.

CLINICAL CASE: MAXIMUM ANDROGEN BLOCKADE IN METASTATIC PROSTATE CANCER

Case History:

A 79-year-old male with a new diagnosis of Gleason score 4 + 5 adenocarcinoma of the prostate presents with multiple metastases on the lumbar vertebrae and several radiologically enlarged pelvic lymph nodes and a PSA of 59 ng/ml. He is otherwise asymptomatic. He elects bilateral orchiectomy for androgen deprivation. In this setting, should he also be placed on flutamide for maximal androgen blockade?

Suggested Answer:

This study and current evidence-based guidelines would suggest no substantial benefit to the addition of long-term nonsteroidal anti-androgens such as flutamide. While there may be a potential benefit to antiandrogens in the short term for patients using gonadotropin releasing hormone agonists to prevent a symptom flare, long-term use in this setting in addition to androgen deprivation therapy does not confer a meaningful enough survival benefit to outweigh the increased side effects.

References

1. Eisenberger MA, Blumenstein BA, Crawford ED, et al. Bilateral orchiectomy with or without flutamide for metastatic prostate cancer. *N Engl J Med.* 1998;339(15):1036–42.
2. Crawford ED, Eisenberger MA, McLeod DG, et al. A controlled trial of leuprolide with and without flutamide in prostatic carcinoma. *N Engl J Med.* 1989;321(7):419–24.
3. Prostate Cancer Trialists' Collaborative Group. Maximum androgen blockade in advanced prostate cancer: an overview of the randomised trials. *Lancet.* 2000;355(9214):1491–8.
4. Cornford P, Bellmunt J, Bolla M, et al. EAU-ESTRO-SIOG guidelines on prostate cancer. Part II: treatment of relapsing, metastatic, and castration-resistant prostate cancer. *Eur Urol.* 2017;71(4):630–42.

14

Intermittent Versus Continuous Androgen Deprivation in Prostate Cancer

Intermittent Androgen Deprivation Therapy (SWOG Trial 9346)

NIRANJAN SATHIANATHEN AND PHILIPP DAHM

"Our results failed to show that intermittent therapy was noninferior to continuous therapy with respect to survival."[1]

Research Question: In patients with metastatic, hormone-sensitive prostate cancer, how does intermittent androgen deprivation (IAD) therapy compare to continuous androgen deprivation (CAD)?

Funding: National Cancer Institute, AstraZeneca, Fonds Cancer (FOCA)

Year Study Began: 1995

Year Study Published: 2013

Study Location: Multiple academic centers in various countries

Who Was Studied: Men with newly diagnosed, metastatic, hormone-sensitive prostate cancer with a pretreatment prostate specific antigen (PSA) level over 5 ng/ml and those who had a declining PSA (less than 4 ng/ml) after 7 months of induction treatment with a luteinizing hormone–releasing hormone (LHRH) agonist and an anti-androgen.

Who Was Excluded: Patients who had received more than 4 months of neoadjuvant and/or adjuvant androgen deprivation therapy (ADT); those who did not have a PSA response after 7 months; patients who were planned to receive concomitant chemotherapy, biological response modifiers, or radiation therapy for reasons other than severe pain

Patients: 1,749

Study Overview:

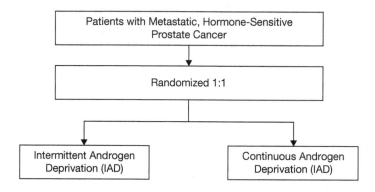

Study Interventions:

- Induction course of a LHRH agonist and an anti-androgen for 7 months in all eligible patients. Men with a PSA response to less than 4 ng/ml were randomized to either IAD or CAD.
- This was a non-inferiority study design with randomization stratified by performance status, prior hormone therapy, and extent of disease.
- Clinical assessments were performed every 3 months and PSA levels measured every month.
- Men in the IAD group stopped androgen ablation therapy at the time of randomization and were recommended to restart when their PSA rose to 20 ng/ml. Investigators were allowed to reinitiate treatment at a PSA of 10 ng/ml at their discretion or when symptoms developed. Reinitiated androgen ablation therapy was then continued for another 7 months and then held if the PSA declined to below 4 ng/ml or continued if it remained above this threshold.
- If the PSA levels rose before the third month of any off-treatment period, treatment was reinitiated and continued until disease progression.

- For patients in the continuous ADT group, treatment was continued from the time of randomization until disease progression.

Follow-up: Median 9.8 years

Endpoints: Overall survival, treatment-specific symptoms (potency, libido, vitality/fatigue), physical functioning, emotional functioning, adverse events, general symptoms, role functioning, global perception of quality of life, social functioning

---

RESULTS:

- The median overall survival in the intermittent ADT group was 5.1 years compared to 5.8 years in the continuous group (hazard ratio [HR] 1.10, 95% confidence interval [CI], 0.99 to 1.23).
- Based on this finding, non-inferiority was not rejected given that the upper limit of the confidence level exceeded the prespecified threshold of 1.20.
- At 15 months, 78% of men in the intermittent group had resumed hormone therapy.
- Predefined subgroup analyses did not suggest any subgroup effects.
- At 3 months, men receiving IAD were less likely to report impotence and had better mental health.
- Outcomes for libido, vitality, and physical functioning favored IAD at 9 and 15 months but did not meet predefined thresholds for statistical significance.

Criticisms and Limitations: This was an open-label study without blinding of patients, personnel, or outcome assessors, which is most relevant to the outcomes other than overall survival. The time periods off ADT may have been short for patients to recover their testosterone level and experience meaningful quality-of-life improvements.

Other Relevant Studies and Information:

- A secondary analysis of this trial linking to Medicare claim data failed to demonstrate a protective effect of IAD against bone loss, metabolic syndrome, and cardiovascular problems and suggested an increased risk of ischemic and thrombotic events (HR 0.69, p = 0.02).[2]

- A recent high-quality systematic review that included 15 trials with biochemically recurrent or metastatic disease found that IAD was not inferior to CAD with respect to overall survival; some quality-of-life criteria seemed improved.[3]
- The topic remains one of considerable controversy as reflected by these contrary editorials.[4,5]

Summary and Implications: This study was the largest study comparing IAD with CAD specific to metastatic disease. Whereas several systematic reviews, typically looking across populations with biochemical recurrence alone and those with metastatic disease, have come to other conclusions, namely that any differences in oncological outcomes can be expected to be small, thereby suggesting non-inferiority,[3,6] its findings have raised caution about the use of IAD in patients with metastatic disease. Quality-of-life and toxicity benefits may only be small. In the current prostate cancer guidelines by the European Urological Association (EAU), CAD remains the standard of care.[7] It suggests that the use of IAD be limited to well-informed, compliant patients who have a good initial PSA response.

CLINICAL CASE: IAD

Case History:

A 73-year-old, otherwise very healthy man presents with newly diagnosed, metastatic, hormone-sensitive prostate cancer following radical prostatectomy 6 years ago and no adjuvant or salvage treatment. He is seeking guidance as to the form of systemic ADT. He is not sexually active and place a high value on maximizing his life expectancy.

Suggested Answer:

In accordance with EAU guidelines and the findings of this study, this patient should be counseled that CAD is currently considered the default management approach in men with metastatic prostate cancer. This will maximize the effect of the systemic ADT. Potential quality-of-life improvements with IAD may be small and the impacts on libido and erectile function appear of secondary importance in him.

References

1. Hussain M, Tangen CM, Berry DL, et al. Intermittent versus continuous androgen deprivation in prostate cancer. *N Engl J Med.* 2013;368(14):1314–25.

2. Hershman DL, Unger JM, Wright JD, et al. Adverse health events following intermittent and continuous androgen deprivation in patients with metastatic prostate cancer. *JAMA Oncol.* 2016;2(4):453–61.

3. Magnan S, Zarychanski R, Pilote L, et al. Intermittent vs. continuous androgen deprivation therapy for prostate cancer: a systematic review and meta-analysis. *JAMA Oncol.* 2015;1(9):1261–9.

4. Klotz L, Higano CS. Intermittent androgen deprivation therapy: an important treatment option for prostate cancer. *JAMA Oncol.* 2016;2(12):1531–2.

5. Hussain M, Tangen C, Higano C, et al. Evaluating intermittent androgen-deprivation therapy phase III clinical trials: the devil is in the details. *J Clin Oncol.* 2016;34(3):280–5.

6. Niraula S, Le LW, Tannock IF. Treatment of prostate cancer with intermittent versus continuous androgen deprivation: a systematic review of randomized trials. *J Clin Oncol.* 2013;31(16):2029–36.

7. Cornford P, Bellmunt J, Bolla M, et al. EAU-ESTRO-SIOG guidelines on prostate cancer. Part II: treatment of relapsing, metastatic, and castration-resistant prostate cancer. *Eur Urol.* 2017;71(4):630–42.

15

Docetaxel Plus Prednisone or Mitoxantrone Plus Prednisone for Advanced Prostate Cancer

The TAX 327 Trial

JOSEPH ZABELL

"Our findings provide evidence that cytotoxic chemotherapy can significantly prolong survival among men with hormone-refractory prostate cancer."[1]

Research Question: In patients with advanced, hormone-refractory prostate cancer, does treatment with docetaxel plus prednisone improve survival?

Funding: Aventis Pharma (now Sanofi)

Year Study Began: 2000

Year Study Published: 2004

Study Location: Sites in 24 countries

Who Was Studied: Patients with histologically or cytologically confirmed adenocarcinoma of the prostate with clinical or radiologic evidence of metastatic disease who had experienced disease progression during hormonal therapy and were receiving primary androgen ablation therapy as maintenance therapy

Who Was Excluded: Men with a Karnofsky performance status score of less than 60% and prior treatment with cytotoxic agents (except estramustine) or radioisotopes

Patients: 1,006

Study Overview:

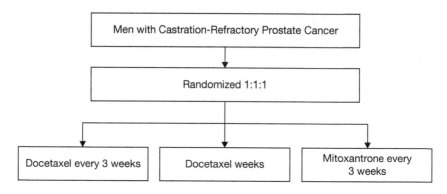

Study Interventions: All men received prednisone 5 mg twice daily. Patients were randomized to three groups:

- 12 mg/m^2 mitoxantrone every 3 weeks
- 75 mg/m^2 docetaxel every 3 weeks
- 30 mg/m^2 docetaxel weekly for 5 of every 6 weeks

Follow-up: Median follow-up of 21 months

Endpoints: Primary outcome: overall survival. Secondary outcomes: reduction in pain (defined as 2-point reduction in Present Pain Intensity [PPI] score without increase in analgesic score, or 50% reduction in analgesic score without increase in PPI score), improvement in quality of life (according to Functional Assessment of Cancer Therapy-Prostate [FACT-P] questionnaire), reduction in serum prostate-specific antigen (PSA) levels of 50%, and objective tumor responses

RESULTS:

- 1,006 patients underwent randomization (335 docetaxel every 3 weeks, 334 weekly docetaxel, 337 mitoxantrone every 3 weeks) (Table 15.1).

- Overall survival
  - Docetaxel every 3 weeks compared to mitoxantrone: hazard ratio (HR) 0.76 (95% confidence interval [CI], 0.62 to 0.94)
  - Docetaxel weekly compared to mitoxantrone: HR 0.91 (95% CI, 0.75 to 1.11)
  - Combined docetaxel groups compared to mitoxantrone: HR 0.83 (95% CI, 0.70 to 0.99; p = 0.04)
- Survival benefit of docetaxel was consistent across subgroups of baseline pain, performance status, and age.
- There was a significant reduction in pain in the group receiving docetaxel every 3 weeks versus mitoxantrone (35% vs. 22%, p = 0.01).
- Quality-of-life improvement was better in the docetaxel groups relative to the mitoxantrone group.
- Overall toxicity rates were low, but the docetaxel groups had a higher incidence of adverse effects.

Table 15.1 SUMMARY OF THE TAX 327 TRIAL

Outcome	Docetaxel Every 3 Weeks	Weekly Docetaxel	Mitoxantrone
Death rate	49.5%	56.9%	59.6%
Median survival	18.9 months	17.4 months	16.5 months
Quality-of-life response rate	22%	23%	13%
>1 serious adverse event	7.8%	8.8%	6.0%

Criticism and Limitations:

- While survival was improved for docetaxel patients, the absolute median survival improvement was less than 3 months.
- The docetaxel groups received twice the dose of steroids that the mitoxantrone group did, which may have improved results in these patients.

Other Relevant Studies and Information:

- SWOG-9916 was another similar study also demonstrating efficacy of docetaxel as first-line treatment in symptomatic metastatic castration-resistant prostate cancer.[2]
- Data from this trial were updated in 2008, demonstrating continued survival benefit for men taking docetaxel, with a median survival time

difference of 2.9 months. In addition, the 3-year survival rate was 18.6% for the patients taking docetaxel every 3 weeks compared with 13.5% for those in the mitoxantrone arm.[3]

- Evidence-based guidelines by the American Urological Association[4] and the European Association of Urology[5] recommend docetaxel as one of several available treatment options for men with asymptomatic, minimally symptomatic, or symptomatic metastatic castration-refractory prostate cancer.

Summary and Implications: This trial served as a landmark study in identifying prostate cancer as a malignancy susceptible to cytotoxic chemotherapy, and its publication was key to the US Food and Drug Administration's approval of docetaxel for use in metastatic castration-refractory prostate cancer, typically with every-3-week dosing. Results have also served as a springboard for additional studies (Chemohormonal Therapy Versus Androgen Ablation Randomized Trial for Extensive Disease in Prostate Cancer [CHAARTED][6] and Systemic Therapy in Advancing or Metastatic Prostate Cancer: Evaluation of Drug Efficacy [STAMPEDE][7]) that have identified docetaxel's efficacy in hormone-sensitive metastatic prostate cancer and continued to expand indications for this agent in the treatment of prostate cancer.

CLINICAL CASE: DOCETAXEL PLUS PREDNISONE OR MITOXANTRONE PLUS PREDNISONE FOR ADVANCED PROSTATE CANCER

Case History:
A 79-year-old male presents with Gleason score 4 + 5 adenocarcinoma of the prostate with multiple metastases on the lumbar vertebrae and several radiologically enlarged pelvic and retroperitoneal lymph nodes and a PSA of 109 ng/ml. He is initially treated with androgen deprivation with PSA response, but now develops a rising PSA and worsening bone pain. Based on the results of this study, is docetaxel a reasonable treatment option? What improvements might the patient experience while on this treatment?

Suggested Answer:
The current study suggests that there is an overall survival benefit to using docetaxel in this setting, particularly if the patient has a good performance status. In addition to the survival benefit, patients receiving docetaxel therapy may experience reductions in pain and improvements in quality of life.

References

1. Tannock IF, de Wit R, Berry WR, et al. Docetaxel plus prednisone or mitoxantrone plus prednisone for advanced prostate cancer. *N Engl J Med* 2004;351(15):1502–12. doi: 10.1056/NEJMoa040720

2. Petrylak DP, Tangen CM, Hussain MH, et al. Docetaxel and estramustine compared with mitoxantrone and prednisone for advanced refractory prostate cancer. *N Engl J Med* 2004;351(15):1513–20. doi: 10.1056/NEJMoa041318

3. Berthold DR, Pond GR, Soban F, et al. Docetaxel plus prednisone or mitoxantrone plus prednisone for advanced prostate cancer: updated survival in the TAX 327 study. *J Clin Oncol* 2008;26(2):242–5. doi: 10.1200/JCO.2007.12.4008 [published online first: 2008/01/10]

4. Cookson MS, Lowrance WT, Murad MH, et al. Castration-resistant prostate cancer: AUA guideline amendment. *J Urol* 2015;193(2):491–9. doi: 10.1016/j.juro.2014.10.104 [published online first: 2014/12/03]

5. Cornford P, Bellmunt J, Bolla M, et al. EAU-ESTRO-SIOG guidelines on prostate cancer. Part II: treatment of relapsing, metastatic, and castration-resistant prostate cancer. *Eur Urol* 2017;71(4):630–42. doi: 10.1016/j.eururo.2016.08.002 [published online first: 2016/09/07]

6. Sweeney CJ, Chen YH, Carducci M, et al. Chemohormonal therapy in meta-static hormone-sensitive prostate cancer. *N Engl J Med* 2015;373(8):737–46. doi: 10.1056/NEJMoa1503747

7. James ND, Sydes MR, Clarke NW, et al. Addition of docetaxel, zoledronic acid, or both to first-line long-term hormone therapy in prostate cancer (STAMPEDE): survival results from an adaptive, multiarm, multistage, platform randomised controlled trial. *Lancet* 2016;387(10024):1163–77. doi: 10.1016/S0140-6736(15)01037-5 [published online first: 2016/01/01]

16

Chemohormonal Therapy in Metastatic Hormone-Sensitive Prostate Cancer

The Chemohormonal Therapy Versus Androgen Ablation Randomized Trial for Extensive Disease in Prostate Cancer (CHAARTED) Trial

PHILIPP DAHM

"Six cycles of docetaxel at the beginning of ADT for metastatic prostate cancer resulted in significantly longer overall survival than that with ADT alone."[1]

Research Question: In patients with metastatic, hormone-sensitive prostate cancer, how does concomitant docetaxel therapy plus systemic androgen deprivation therapy (ADT) compare to ADT alone?

Funding: National Cancer Institute and Sanofi

Year Study Began: July 2006

Year Study Published: August 2015

Study Location: Multiple institutions in the United States

Who Was Studied: Men with a diagnosis of prostate cancer, documented metastatic disease, and good performance status

Who Was Excluded: Patients with poor renal or hepatic function and those who had received systemic ADT for longer than 120 days

Patients: 790

Study Overview:

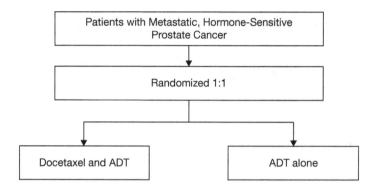

Study Interventions: Patients in the intervention arm received systemic ADT plus docetaxel at a dose of 75 mg/m² every 3 weeks for six cycles, with premedication with 8 mg oral dexamethasone at 12 hours, 3 hours, and 1 hour before docetaxel infusion. Patients in the control arm received ADT only. In both arms ADT was achieved by either luteinizing hormone–releasing hormone (LHRH) agonist therapy, LHRH antagonist therapy, or surgical castration. In the docetaxel-plus-ADT arm up to two dose modifications could be made for toxicity; these patients were seen every 3 weeks, whereas patients in the ADT arm were only seen every 3 months. Prostate-specific antigen (PSA) levels were assessed at each scheduled visit. Imaging such as computed tomography scans and bone scans were obtained at baseline, at the time of development of castration resistance, and when clinically indicated.

Follow-up: Median follow-up for both groups was approximately 29 months.

Endpoints: Primary outcome: overall survival. Secondary outcomes included time to clinical progression (radiographic or symptomatic deterioration due to disease), time to development of hormone-refractory disease, time to serological progression, frequency of adverse events, and the tolerability of chemotherapy.

RESULTS:

- The mean patient age was 64 years and the median PSA was around 50 ng/ml.
- Approximately two-thirds of patents had an Eastern Cooperative Oncology Group (ECOG) performance status of 0, and two-thirds of patients had a high volume of metastases (four or more bone lesions and at least one lesion beyond vertebral bodies and pelvis).
- Median overall survival was 13.6 months longer with ADT plus docetaxel (combination therapy) than with ADT alone (57.6 months vs. 44.0 months; hazard ratio [HR] 0.61; 95% confidence interval [CI], 0.47 to 0.80).
- The median time to progression was 20.2 months in the combination group versus 11.7 months in the ADT-alone group (HR 0.61; 95% CI, 0.51 to 0.72).
- In the combination group, the rate of grade 3 or 4 febrile neutropenia was 6.2%, the rate of grade 3 or 4 infection with neutropenia was 2.3%, and the rate of grade 3 sensory neuropathy and of grade 3 motor neuropathy was 0.5%. None of these types of adverse events occurred in the ADT-alone arm.

Criticism and Limitations: Two post hoc protocol revisions impacted the validity of the study results, namely the sample size increase to account for better-than-expected survival in the control group and the expanded inclusion of initially only patients with high-volume disease to also include those with low-volume disease. The results for the latter smaller group were not statistically significant, thereby raising a question about a subgroup effect.

Other Relevant Studies and Information:

- Quality-of-life data from this trial have since been reported separately.[2] There may be a small but clinically unimportant improvement in quality of life with combination therapy.
- The Genitourinary Group of the Association Française (GETUG-AFU)-15 was a similar yet smaller study of early chemohormonal therapy that failed to demonstrate a benefit.[3]
- Systemic Therapy in Advancing or Metastatic Prostate Cancer: Evaluation of Drug Efficacy (STAMPEDE), a three-armed trial that included a comparison of early combination therapy versus ADT alone, also demonstrated a survival benefit.[4]

- A individual patient meta-analysis of all three trials[5] and a Cochrane review[6] indicate that the addition of taxane-based chemotherapy to ADT for hormone-sensitive prostate cancer probably prolongs both overall and disease-specific survival and delays disease progression but comes with an increase in toxicity.

Summary and Implications: Based on the results of this trial, initial treatment with chemotherapy is now an option in the treatment algorithm for men with newly diagnosed metastatic prostate cancer, in particular for those with high-volume disease.

CLINICAL CASE: UPFRONT DOCETAXEL-BASED CHEMOTHERAPY IN NEWLY DIAGNOSED HORMONE-SENSITIVE PROSTATE CANCER

Case History:

A 75-year-old patient is noted to have a PSA level of 250 ng/ml and is diagnosed with Gleason score 4 + 5 adenocarcinoma of the prostate with widespread bone metastases to the vertebral column, ribs, and skull as well as widespread pelvic lymphadenopathy. He is started on bicalutamide and administered a first injection of leuprolide. Would he benefit from the addition of early docetaxel-based chemotherapy?

Suggested Answer:

Current evidence-based guidelines recommend castration combined with docetaxel as the standard of care in patients with newly diagnosed prostate cancer, assuming the patient is fit enough to undergo chemotherapy.[7] This is least controversial in a patient like the one in this scenario with a high burden of disease who is likely to derive survival benefit in absolute terms. Expected side effects are mainly hematological in nature in the form of asymptomatic and febrile neutropenia.

References

1. Sweeney CJ, Chen YH, Carducci M, et al. Chemohormonal therapy in metastatic hormone-sensitive prostate cancer. *N Engl J Med.* 2015;373(8):737–46.
2. Morgans AK, Chen YH, Sweeney CJ, et al. Quality of life during treatment with chemohormonal therapy: analysis of E3805 chemohormonal androgen ablation randomized trial in prostate cancer. *J Clin Oncol.* 2018;36(11):1088–95.

3. Gravis G, Fizazi K, Joly F, et al. Androgen-deprivation therapy alone or with docetaxel in non-castrate metastatic prostate cancer (GETUG-AFU 15): a randomised, open-label, phase 3 trial. *Lancet Oncol.* 2013;14(2):149–58.

4. James ND, Sydes MR, Clarke NW, et al. Addition of docetaxel, zoledronic acid, or both to first-line long-term hormone therapy in prostate cancer (STAMPEDE): survival results from an adaptive, multiarm, multistage, platform randomised controlled trial. *Lancet.* 2016;387(10024):1163–77.

5. Vale CL, Burdett S, Rydzewska LHM, et al. Addition of docetaxel or bisphosphonates to standard of care in men with localised or metastatic, hormone-sensitive prostate cancer: a systematic review and meta-analyses of aggregate data. *Lancet Oncol.* 2016;17(2):243–56.

6. Sathianathen NJ, Philippou YA, Kuntz GM, et al. Taxane-based chemohormonal therapy for metastatic hormone-sensitive prostate cancer. *Cochrane Database Syst Rev.* 2018;10:CD012816.

7. Cornford P, Bellmunt J, Bolla M, et al. EAU-ESTRO-SIOG guidelines on prostate cancer. Part II: treatment of relapsing, metastatic, and castration-resistant prostate cancer. *Eur Urol.* 2017;71(4):630–42.

17

Abiraterone and Increased Survival in Metastatic Prostate Cancer

JOSEPH ZABELL

"The inhibition of androgen biosynthesis by abiraterone acetate prolonged overall survival among patients with metastatic castration-resistant prostate cancer who previously received chemotherapy."[1]

Research Question: In patients with castration-resistant prostate cancer who have received prior chemotherapy, does abiraterone acetate, an inhibitor of androgen biosynthesis, compared to placebo prolong survival?

Funding: Cougar Biotechnology

Year Study Began: 2008

Year Study Published: 2011

Study Location: Multinational study at 147 sites in 13 countries

Who Was Studied: Men with histologically or cytologically confirmed prostate cancer who had previously been treated with docetaxel, with disease progression (two consecutive increases in prostate-specific antigen [PSA]) or radiographic progression, and ongoing androgen deprivation

Who Was Excluded: Men with liver metastases or abnormal liver enzymes or those with previous therapy with ketoconazole

Patients: 1,195

Study Overview:

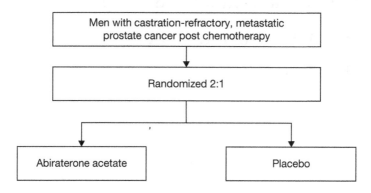

Study Interventions: Patients received 1 g abiraterone acetate or placebo once daily. All patients received prednisone 5 mg orally twice daily.

Follow-up: Median follow-up was 12.8 months.

Endpoints: Primary outcome: overall survival. Secondary outcomes: time to PSA progression (defined as at least 50% of pretreatment PSA level), radiologic evidence of progression-free survival, response according to Response Evaluation Criteria in Solid Tumors (RECIST).

RESULTS:

- 1,195 patients underwent randomization (797 to abiraterone and 398 to placebo).
- Overall survival was longer in the abiraterone group (14.8 months) than in the placebo group (10.9 months) (hazard ratio 0.65; 95% confidence interval, 0.54 to 0.77; p < 0.001).
- Time to PSA progression was longer in the abiraterone group (10.2 vs. 6.6 months; p < 0.001).
- Progression-free survival was longer in the abiraterone group (5.6 vs. 3.6 months; p < 0.001).

- PSA response rate was better in the abiraterone group (29% vs. 6%; p < 0.001).
- The most common adverse events were fatigue, back pain, nausea, constipation, bone pain, and arthralgia. Adverse events leading to treatment discontinuation and dose modification were similar in the two groups.
- Toxic effects related to mineralocorticoid excess resulting from blockade of CYP17 included hypokalemia, hypertension, and fluid retention; were mostly grade 1 or 2; and were mitigated by prednisolone.

Criticism and Limitations: The study did not fully discuss the degree of treatment compliance or crossover. It also did not report on the type of treatments received after progression, which may have biased outcomes. The study was funded and overseen by the sponsor company and the analysis was performed and the manuscript written—at least in part—by employees of the sponsor. It was stopped early for benefit after a planned interim analysis, a practice that may potentially result in an overestimate of the true effect size.[2]

Other Relevant Studies and Information:

- Abiraterone with prednisone has demonstrated clinical efficacy and improved survival in the pre- and post-docetaxel setting for patients with metastatic castration-resistant prostate cancer (mCRPC).[3,4]
- American Urological Association[5] and European Association of Urology[6] guidelines recommend abiraterone plus prednisone as one of several available treatment options for men with asymptomatic or minimally symptomatic mCRPC with good performance status both before and after docetaxel chemotherapy.

Summary and Implications: Docetaxel represented one of the earliest systemic agents to demonstrate survival benefits for patients with mCRPC.[7] In the setting of mCRPC with progression following docetaxel chemotherapy, this study of abiraterone with prednisone prolonged overall survival and provided benefits in multiple secondary endpoints over placebo.[1] This study expedited the use of this relatively well-tolerated agent in the post-chemotherapy setting and set the stage for subsequent trials that have moved the use of abiraterone into the pre-chemotherapy setting.[4] These trials have also demonstrated improvements in overall and progression-free survival with the use of abiraterone in chemotherapy-naïve patients with mCRPC.[3,4]

CLINICAL CASE: ABIRATERONE FOLLOWING DOCETAXEL-BASED CHEMOTHERAPY

Case History:

A 79-year-old male with a history of Gleason score 4 + 5 adenocarcinoma of the prostate presents with multiple apparent metastases on the lumbar vertebrae and several radiologically enlarged pelvic lymph nodes. He has previously been treated with androgen deprivation therapy and remains on leuprolide. He ultimately demonstrated evidence of progression and received docetaxel chemotherapy. Following chemotherapy, he has now noted subsequent PSA rises over the past 6 months. Would abiraterone be an appropriate option in this clinical scenario?

Suggested Answer:

Based on current, evidence-based guidelines founded on this trial, this patient would be a good candidate for abiraterone plus prednisone, assuming good overall performance status. This trial suggests benefits in terms of overall survival as well as time to PSA progression and progression-free survival in these patients.

References

1. de Bono JS, Logothetis CJ, Molina A, et al. Abiraterone and increased survival in metastatic prostate cancer. *N Engl J Med* 2011;364(21):1995–2005. doi: 10.1056/NEJMoa1014618
2. Bassler D, Briel M, Montori VM, et al. Stopping randomized trials early for benefit and estimation of treatment effects: systematic review and meta-regression analysis. *JAMA* 2010;303(12):1180–7. doi: 10.1001/jama.2010.310 [published online first: 2010/03/25]
3. Ryan CJ, Smith MR, de Bono JS, et al. Abiraterone in metastatic prostate cancer without previous chemotherapy. *N Engl J Med* 2013;368(2):138–48. doi: 10.1056/NEJMoa1209096 [published online first: 2012/12/12]
4. Ryan CJ, Smith MR, Fizazi K, et al. Abiraterone acetate plus prednisone versus placebo plus prednisone in chemotherapy-naive men with metastatic castration-resistant prostate cancer (COU-AA-302): final overall survival analysis of a randomised, double-blind, placebo-controlled phase 3 study. *Lancet Oncol* 2015;16(2):152–60. doi: 10.1016/S1470-2045(14)71205-7 [published online first: 2015/01/21]

5. Cookson MS, Lowrance WT, Murad MH, et al. Castration-resistant prostate cancer: AUA guideline amendment. *J Urol* 2015;193(2):491–9. doi: 10.1016/j.juro.2014.10.104 [published online first: 2014/12/03]

6. Cornford P, Bellmunt J, Bolla M, et al. EAU-ESTRO-SIOG guidelines on prostate cancer. Part II: treatment of relapsing, metastatic, and castration-resistant prostate cancer. *Eur Urol* 2017;71(4):630–42. doi: 10.1016/j.eururo.2016.08.002 [published online first: 2016/09/07]

7. Tannock IF, de Wit R, Berry WR, et al. Docetaxel plus prednisone or mitoxantrone plus prednisone for advanced prostate cancer. *N Engl J Med* 2004;351(15):1502–12. doi: 10.1056/NEJMoa040720

18

Enzalutamide in Metastatic Prostate Cancer Before Chemotherapy

The PREVAIL Study

JOSEPH ZABELL

"Enzalutamide significantly decreased the risk of radiographic progression and death and delayed the initiation of chemotherapy in men with metastatic prostate cancer."[1]

Research Question: In men with metastatic castration-resistant prostate cancer (mCRPC), does enzalutamide, an oral androgen-receptor inhibitor, prolong survival when administered prior to chemotherapy?

Funding: Medivation and Astellas Pharma

Year Study Began: 2010

Year Study Published: 2014

Study Location: Multinational study at 207 sites

Who Was Studied: Men with histologically or cytologically confirmed adenocarcinoma of the prostate with documented metastases and prostate-specific antigen (PSA) progression, radiographic progression, or both in bone or soft tissue, despite receiving luteinizing hormone–releasing hormone (LHRH) analog therapy or undergoing orchiectomy. Continued androgen deprivation was required.

Who Was Excluded: Men with an Eastern Cooperative Oncology Group (ECOG) performance status greater than 1 and those who had previously received cytotoxic agents (except estramustine) or radioisotopes

Patients: 1,717

Study Overview:

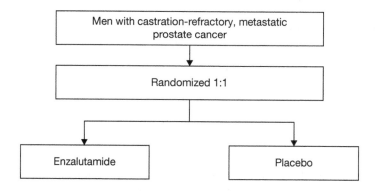

Study Interventions: Men received either daily enzalutamide 160 mg or placebo.

Follow-up: Median follow-up of 22 months

Endpoints: Co-primary outcomes: overall survival and radiographic progression-free survival. Secondary outcomes: time to initiation of cytotoxic chemotherapy, time until first skeletal-related event, best overall soft-tissue response, time to PSA progression, and decline in PSA level of 50% or more from baseline.

RESULTS:

- Overall survival: The hazard ratio (HR) for time to death was 0.71 (95% confidence interval [CI], 0.60 to 0.84) in favor of enzalutamide. Median overall survival time was estimated at 32.4 months for the enzalutamide group and 30.2 months for the placebo group.
- For radiographic progression-free survival, the HR was 0.19 (95% CI, 0.15 to 0.23) favoring enzalutamide.

- Enzalutamide provided prolonged time to cytotoxic chemotherapy (28.0 months enzalutamide vs. 10.8 months for placebo; HR 0.35; p < 0.001).
- Enzalutamide prolonged time until first skeletal-related event (HR 0.72; p < 0.001).
- The enzalutamide group had improved complete or partial soft-tissue response (59% vs. 5%; p < 0.001).
- Subsequent antineoplastic agents were received by 40% of the patients in the enzalutamide group and 70% of those in the placebo group.
- Serious (grade 3 or higher) adverse events were reported in 43% of those in the enzalutamide group and 37% of those in the placebo group. Median time to severe adverse event was 22.3 months for the enzalutamide group and 13.3 months for the placebo group. Fatigue and hypertension were the most common clinically relevant adverse events.

Criticism and Limitations: The study did not fully report the degree of treatment compliance and/or crossover, nor did it provide details about subsequent secondary treatment after progression occurred (and its potential impact on outcomes). Despite a very large relative effect size, absolute effect sizes (in terms of months of life gained) were relatively modest. The study was stopped early for benefit, resulting in reduced precision (wider confidence intervals) and potential bias.[2]

Other Relevant Studies and Information:

- The authors of the PREVAIL study, which was stopped early for benefit, subsequently reported an extended analysis, which confirmed its findings.[3]
- A prior study had demonstrated that enzalutamide improves survival in the post-docetaxel stage for men with mCRPC.[4]

Summary and Implications: Docetaxel was the earliest systemic agents to demonstrate survival benefits for patients with mCRPC.[6] Since then, a number of agents have become available for use either before or after the administration of chemotherapy. Enzalutamide, an androgen receptor–signaling inhibitor that binds to the androgen receptor with a higher affinity than bicalutamide, inhibits androgen receptor translocation, and has reduced agonist activity when compared with standard anti-androgens, is one such agent.[7] Enzalutamide was approved by the US Food and Drug Administration in 2012 and was initially demonstrated to have survival benefit in the post-chemotherapy state in the AFFIRM study.[4] The current study by Beer et al. expanded the indication for enzalutamide into the pre-chemotherapy disease state given the benefits of this agent in terms of overall and radiographic progression-free survival. Based largely on the results in this randomized clinical trial, recent evidence-based guidelines by the American Urological Association (AUA)[5] and the European Association of Urology (EAU)[6] currently recommend enzalutamide as one of several available agents for men with asymptomatic or minimally symptomatic mCRPC with good performance status and no prior docetaxel chemotherapy.

CLINICAL CASE: ENZALUTAMIDE FOR MCRPC

Case History:

A 72-year-old male presents with a history of prostate cancer after undergoing radical prostatectomy 5 years earlier. Pathology at that time demonstrated Gleason 4 + 5 disease with extracapsular extension, positive margins, and positive pelvic lymph nodes. He has been on systemic androgen deprivation therapy (ADT) since that time with several years of good PSA control but now presents with rising PSA and evidence of new yet asymptomatic metastatic lesions detected on a bone scan. Based on the results of this trial, would enzalutamide be appropriate for this patient?

Suggested Answer:

Based on evidence from this trial and in accordance with current AUA and EAU guidelines, this patient would be a candidate for enzalutamide therapy assuming he has good overall performance status. This would be administered once daily. Current guidelines recommend the use of this enzalutamide in this disease space as it has demonstrated improvement in overall and radiographic progression-free survival for those who receive it prior to chemotherapy.

References

1. Beer TM, Armstrong AJ, Rathkopf DE, et al. Enzalutamide in metastatic prostate cancer before chemotherapy. *N Engl J Med* 2014;371(5):424–33. doi: 10.1056/ NEJMoa1405095

2. Bassler D, Montori VM, Briel M, et al. Early stopping of randomized clinical trials for overt efficacy is problematic. *J Clin Epidemiol* 2008;61(3):241–6. doi: 10.1016/ j.jclinepi.2007.07.016 [published online first: 2008/01/30]

3. Beer TM, Armstrong AJ, Rathkopf D, et al. Enzalutamide in men with chemotherapy-naive metastatic castration-resistant prostate cancer: extended analysis of the phase

3 PREVAIL study. *Eur Urol* 2017;71(2):151–4. doi: 10.1016/j.eururo.2016.07.032 [published online first: 2016/08/02]

4. Scher HI, Fizazi K, Saad F, et al. Increased survival with enzalutamide in prostate cancer after chemotherapy. *N Engl J Med* 2012;367(13):1187–97. doi: 10.1056/NEJMoa1207506 [published online first: 2012/08/17]

5. Cookson MS, Lowrance WT, Murad MH, et al. Castration-resistant prostate cancer: AUA guideline amendment. *J Urol* 2015;193(2):491–9. doi: 10.1016/j.juro.2014.10.104 [published online first: 2014/12/03]

6. Cornford P, Bellmunt J, Bolla M, et al. EAU-ESTRO-SIOG guidelines on prostate cancer. Part II: treatment of relapsing, metastatic, and castration-resistant prostate cancer. *Eur Urol* 2017;71(4):630–42. doi: 10.1016/j.eururo.2016.08.002 [published online first: 2016/09/07]

19

The EORTC Intergroup Phase 3 Study Comparing the Oncological Outcome of Elective Nephron-Sparing Surgery and Radical Nephrectomy for Low-Stage Renal Cell Carcinoma

CHRISTOPHER WEIGHT

"Both [nephron-sparing surgery and radical nephrectomy] . . . provide excellent oncologic results."[1]

Research Question: In patients with small renal masses, how does nephron-sparing surgery (NSS) compare to radical nephrectomy (RN)?

Funding: National Cancer Institute (USA) and Fonds Cancer (Belgium)

Year Study Began: 1992

Year Study Published: 2007

Study Location: Numerous sites in Europe and North America

Who Was studied: Patients with a solitary, renal masses less than or equal to 5 cm in largest diameter without invasion of the perinephric fat and a World Health Organization (WHO) performance status of 0 to 2

Who Was excluded: Patients with a solitary kidney, von Hippel–Lindau disease, multifocal disease, T3-T4 tumors, clinical presence of distant or lymphatic metastases, a WHO performance status of more than 2, and another carcinoma, except for adequately treated non-melanoma skin cancer

Patients: 541

Study Overview:

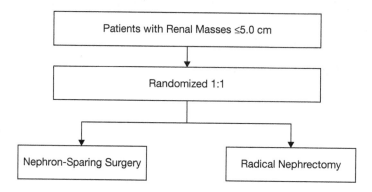

Study Interventions: Patients with small renal masses were centrally randomized to either NSS or RN. Allowable techniques for NSS were tumor excavation (but not enucleation), wedge resection, or partial nephrectomy together with limited lymphadenectomy. Hilar clamping was not routinely done. RN consisted of removal of the entire kidney with the adrenal and perinephric fat with Gerota's fascia intact. Limited lymphadenectomy could be done separately or en bloc and included the lymphatic tissue in the renal hilum and the nodes around the vena cava at the level of the renal veins on the right side and on the aorta at the level of the artery on the left side.[2]

Follow-up: Median of 9.3 years

Endpoints: Primary outcome: overall survival. Secondary outcomes: cancer-specific survival, time to progression, treatment-related complications, and postoperative renal function. A preplanned secondary analysis compared outcomes in those who had pathologically confirmed kidney cancer. The study had a non-inferiority design.

RESULTS:

- Median patient age was approximately 62 years, and two-thirds were male. Less than 40% of participants reported any chronic disease.
- Overall survival favored RN with a hazard ratio (HR) of 1.50 (95% confidence interval, 1.03 to 2.16), with 10-year survival rates of 75.7% for NSS and 81.1% for RN. Only 12 of the 117 deaths were from kidney cancer.
- Progression-free survival was similar for both groups with an HR of 1.37 (95% CI, 0.58 to 3.24); 10-year progression rates were 4.1% for NSS and 3.3% for RN.
- In a predefined subset analysis that excluded patients with non-renal cell carcinoma, the difference in overall survival was less (HR 1.43).
- Severe blood loss (more than 1 liter) was reported in 3.1% of NSS and 1.2% of RN patients. 10 patients (4.4%) in the NSS group developed urinary fistulas.

Criticisms and Limitations: The study was based on unrealistic assumptions with regard to the acceptable margin of non-inferiority of 10% (which was then revised to 3%) and also fell far short of its accrual goal of 1,300 patients. A relatively large proportion of patients (9.8%) were lost to follow-up, raising concern about attrition bias. In addition, 150 patients (27.7%) did not meet the intended study inclusion criteria, nearly half of them (n = 70) because they did not have renal cell carcinoma.

Other Relevant Studies and Information:

- A secondary analysis of participants' long-term renal function found only a small difference in rates of advanced kidney dysfunction (estimated glomerular filtration rate [eGFR] less than 30) of 6.3% after NSS and 10.0% after RN. Rates of kidney failure were similar in both groups at around 1.5%.[3]
- A well-designed observational study of Surveillance, Epidemiology and End Results (SEER) Medicare beneficiaries (n = 7,138) using instrumental variable analysis to adjust for confounding found patients

undergoing partial nephrectomy (PN) to have a lower risk of death compared to RN (HR 0.54; 95% CI, 0.34 to 0.85).[4]
- A systematic review and meta-analysis of PN versus RN that included non-randomized studies found 19% relative risk reduction for all-cause mortality in favor of NSS.[5]
- A Cochrane review rated this study's central finding of worse overall survival in the NSS group as low-quality evidence given issues surrounding study limitations, imprecision, and indirectness (since a large proportion of patients did not actually have a malignant renal mass).[6]
- Current evidence-based guidelines by the American Urological Association and the European Association of Urology favor NSS over RN for small renal masses less than 4 cm, arguing that the risk of chronic kidney disease and its progression may be reduced while oncological outcomes are likely similar.[7,8]

Summary and Implications: This study by the European Organisation for Research and Treatment of Cancer (EORTC) remains the only randomized controlled trial of NSS versus RN, and its findings were quite unexpected. Its finding of decreased overall survival in patients undergoing NSS remains poorly explained and may have been a chance finding (type I statistical error). Its main contribution to the literature has been to suggest that the assumed benefits of NSS over RN based on non-randomized studies may have been drastically overstated and that in most cases RN and PN have comparable outcomes.

CLINICAL CASE: TREATMENT FOR A SMALL RENAL MASS

Case History:
A 60-year-old woman is diagnosed with 4.1-cm exophytic renal mass in her right kidney and a normal contralateral kidney. She undergoes a biopsy and is found to have clear cell kidney cancer. She is otherwise healthy, has not previously had surgery, and also has a normal contralateral kidney. According to this trial, should she undergo RN or PN?

Suggested Answer:
Based on current guidelines,[7,8] this patient should be offered PN, now most commonly performed robotically. This approach likely offers equivalent oncological outcomes but is likely to preserve her current kidney function. The tradeoff for her to consider is an increased risk of bleeding complications and the development of a urinary leak requiring secondary measures.

References

1. Van Poppel H, Da Pozzo L, Albrecht W, et al. A prospective, randomised EORTC intergroup phase 3 study comparing the oncologic outcome of elective nephron-sparing surgery and radical nephrectomy for low-stage renal cell carcinoma. *Eur Urol* 2011;59(4):543–52. doi: 10.1016/j.eururo.2010.12.013 [published online first: 2010/12/28]
2. Van Poppel H, Da Pozzo L, Albrecht W, et al. A prospective randomized EORTC intergroup phase 3 study comparing the complications of elective nephron-sparing surgery and radical nephrectomy for low-stage renal cell carcinoma. *Eur Urol* 2007;51(6):1606–15. doi: 10.1016/j.eururo.2006.11.013 [published online first: 2006/12/05]
3. Scosyrev E, Messing EM, Sylvester R, et al. Renal function after nephron-sparing surgery versus radical nephrectomy: results from EORTC randomized trial 30904. *Eur Urol* 2014;65(2):372–7. doi: 10.1016/j.eururo.2013.06.044 [published online first: 2013/07/16]
4. Tan HJ, Norton EC, Ye Z, et al. Long-term survival following partial vs. radical nephrectomy among older patients with early-stage kidney cancer. *JAMA* 2012;307(15):1629–35. doi: 10.1001/jama.2012.475
5. Kim SP, Thompson RH, Boorjian SA, et al. Comparative effectiveness for survival and renal function of partial and radical nephrectomy for localized renal tumors: a systematic review and meta-analysis. *J Urol* 2012;188(1):51–7. doi: 10.1016/j.juro.2012.03.006 [published online first: 2012/05/18]
6. Kunath F, Schmidt S, Krabbe LM, et al. Partial nephrectomy versus radical nephrectomy for clinical localised renal masses. *Cochrane Database Syst Rev* 2017;5:CD012045. doi: 10.1002/14651858.CD012045.pub2 [published online first: 2017/05/10]
7. Ljungberg B, Albiges L, Bensalah K, et al. Renal cell carcinoma. European Association of Urology; 2019. Available from: https://uroweb.org/guideline/renal-cell-carcinoma/?type=summary-of-changes, accessed 1/13/2020.
8. Campbell S, Uzzo RG, Allaf ME, et al. Renal mass and localized renal cancer: AUA guideline. *J Urol* 2017;198(3):520–9. doi: 10.1016/j.juro.2017.04.100 [published online first: 2017/05/10]

20

Nephrectomy Followed by Interferon Alfa-2b Compared With Interferon Alfa-2b Alone for Metastatic Renal Cell Cancer

CHRISTOPHER WEIGHT

"Nephrectomy followed by interferon therapy results in longer survival among patients with metastatic renal-cell cancer than does interferon therapy alone."[1]

Research Question: In patients with metastatic renal cell carcinoma (RCC), how does nephrectomy followed by alfa interferon-2b compare to alfa interferon-2b alone?

Funding: National Cancer Institute (United States)

Year Study Began: 1989

Year Study Published: 2001

Study Location: 80 sites in the United States as part of the Southwest Oncology Group (SWOG)

Who Was Studied: Men and women over age 18 with a good performance status who had biopsy-confirmed, metastatic clear cell RCC beyond the regional lymph nodes and had not received prior systematic therapy

Who Was Excluded: Patients with a performance status less than 1 based on SWOG criteria and those not deemed to be surgical candidates for radical nephrectomy

Patients: 241

Study Overview:

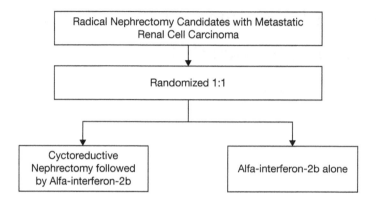

Study Interventions: Patients in the intervention arm underwent radical nephrectomy within 4 weeks of enrollment followed by interferon alfa-2b. Induction interferon therapy was begun at 1.25 million IU/m^2, with escalation to a starting dose of 5 million IU/m^2 on the first day of treatment (1.25 million IU/m^2 3 days before, 2.5 million IU/m^2 2 days before, and 3.75 million IU/m^2 the day before treatment). Interferon was continued 3 days a week at a dose of 5 million IU/m^2 until disease progression. Patients in the control arm were only treated with systemic interferon alfa-2b therapy using the same dose regimen. Patients in both groups were then followed with imaging studies at regular intervals.

Follow-up: Median follow-up was approximately 12 months.

Endpoints: Primary outcome: overall survival. Secondary outcomes: tumor response and adverse events.

RESULTS:

- The mean patient age was approximately 59 years. Over two-thirds were men and a similar proportion had lung metastases only.
- The overall survival was 3 months longer with nephrectomy plus interferon alfa (11.1 months vs. 8.1 months in the group receiving only

interferon alfa) (p = 0.05). Survival at 1 year was 49.7% versus 36.8% (p = 0.012), favoring the cytoreductive nephrectomy group.
- The objective response rates were similar between the two groups: 3.3% for the group receiving cytoreductive nephrectomy plus interferon versus 3.6% for the interferon-only group.
- Subgroup analyses indicated a potentially greater benefit in patients with a more favorable performance status (0 vs. 1) and those with lung metastases only (lung only vs. other).
- 22 patients had surgical complications, including one death after dehiscence, two myocardial infarctions, two wound infections, and a case of severe hypotension. 10 patients had severe complications due to interferon in the cytoreductive-plus-interferon group versus 13 in the interferon only cohort.

Criticism and Limitations: The study only enrolled patients with a good performance status who were surgical candidates for nephrectomy, which limits generalizability. A relatively large proportion of patients (17/120; 14.1%) randomized to the cytoreductive group did not undergo surgery for a variety of reasons but were included in the intention-to-treat analyses, potentially biasing the results toward showing no difference. The p-value for the primary analyses was 0.05, thereby not meeting the investigators' predefined alpha of 0.05, and the reported survival benefit of 3 months was relatively small.

Other Relevant Studies and Information:

- A similar but much smaller study from Europe found a larger, 10-month benefit in median survival in favor of cytoreductive nephrectomy prior to cytokine therapy versus cytokine therapy alone.[2]
- The Cancer du Rein Metastatique Nephrectomie et Antiangiogéniques (CARMENA) trial[3] has since randomized suitable candidates for nephrectomy to undergo nephrectomy and then receive sunitinib (standard therapy) or to receive sunitinib alone. The results in the sunitinib-alone group were non-inferior to those in the nephrectomy-plus-sunitinib group with regard to overall survival (hazard ratio [HR] 0.89; 95% confidence interval [CI], 0.71 to 1.10). The median overall survival was 18.4 months in the sunitinib-alone group and 13.9 months in the nephrectomy-plus-sunitinib group.
- The Immediate Surgery or Surgery After Sunitinib Malate in Treating Patients with Kidney Cancer (SURTIME) trial compared immediate

cytoreductive nephrectomy followed by sunitinib versus cytoreductive nephrectomy after three 6-week courses of sunitinib. Overall survival favored delayed cytoreductive nephrectomy (median 32.4 months) compared with immediate cytoreductive nephrectomy (median 15.1 months) (HR 0.57; 95% CI, 0.34 to 0.95).

Summary and Implications: This trial was the first randomized trial of cytoreductive nephrectomy prior to immunotherapy with alfa interferon-2b, suggesting a modest survival benefit of cytoreductive nephrectomy in patients with a good performance status, in particular those with a low disease burden. These results have long been extrapolated to also apply to the era of targeted therapy until this paradigm was drawn into question by the CARMENA trial. This study has been criticized for its small sample size and non-inferiority design, which may have contributed to its negative findings.

CLINICAL CASE: CYTOREDUCTIVE NEPHRECTOMY

Case History:

A 45-year-old female is diagnosed with large 12-cm right renal mass confirmed to be clear cell carcinoma based on renal biopsy. She also has two approximately 2-cm lung nodules as the only documented sites of metastases. She is otherwise healthy with an excellent performance status. Should she undergo cytoreductive nephrectomy prior to systemic therapy with sunitinib?

Suggested Answer:

Results of this trial, which preceded the era of targeted therapy, indicate a benefit of cytoreductive nephrectomy that the highly controversial CARMENA trial has drawn into question.[3] European Association of Urology guidelines limit the role for cytoreductive nephrectomy (weak recommendation) to those at good risk who may not require immediate systemic therapy or those with oligometastases in whom all metastatic sites can be removed surgically, as in this patient.[4] The patient's young age and low perioperative risk also point toward a more aggressive upfront approach.

References

1. Flanigan RC, Salmon SE, Blumenstein BA, et al. Nephrectomy followed by interferon alfa-2b compared with interferon alfa-2b alone for metastatic renal-cell cancer. *N Engl J Med.* 2001;345(23):1655–9.

2. Mickisch GH, Garin A, van Poppel H, et al. Radical nephrectomy plus interferon-alfa-based immunotherapy compared with interferon alfa alone in metastatic renal-cell carcinoma: a randomised trial. *Lancet.* 2001;358(9286):966–70.

3. Mejean A, Ravaud A, Thezenas S, et al. Sunitinib alone or after nephrectomy in metastatic renal-cell carcinoma. *N Engl J Med.* 2018;379(5):417–27.

4. Ljungberg B, Albiges L, Bensalah K, et al. Renal cell carcinoma: EAU guidelines. Available at: https://uroweb.org/guideline/renal-cell-carcinoma/?type=summary-of-changes. Published 2019. Accessed 1/13/2020.

21

Sunitinib Versus Interferon Alfa in Metastatic Renal Cell Carcinoma

CHRISTOPHER WEIGHT

"Progression-free survival was longer and response rates were higher in patients with metastatic renal-cell cancer who received sunitinib than in those receiving interferon alfa."[1]

Research Question: In patients with previously untreated metastatic renal cell carcinoma (RCC), how does sunitinib compare to interferon alfa?

Funding: Pfizer (USA)

Year Study Began: 2004

Year Study Published: 2007

Study Location: 101 sites in North America, Europe, Australia, and South America.

Who Was Studied: Men and women over the age of 18 with metastatic clear cell RCC. Patients could not have received prior systemic treatment for RCC and had to have an Eastern Cooperative Oncology Group (ECOG) performance status of 0 or 1 and adequate hematologic, coagulation, hepatic, renal, and cardiac function.

Who Was Excluded: Those with brain metastases, uncontrolled hypertension, or clinically significant cardiovascular events or disease during the preceding 12 months

Patients: 750

Study Overview:

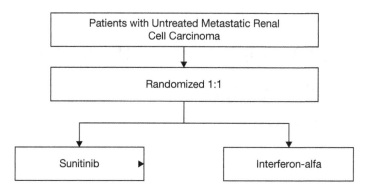

Study Interventions: Patients with previously untreated metastatic clear cell RCC were randomly assigned (in a 1:1 ratio) to receive repeated 6-week cycles of sunitinib 50 mg orally for 4 weeks, followed by 2 weeks without treatment or interferon alfa (9 million units subcutaneously three times a week). The patients were then followed with imaging studies on day 28 of the first four cycles and then every two cycles until the end of treatment.

Follow-up: Median 12 months

Endpoints: Primary outcome: progression-free survival. Secondary outcomes: objective response rate, overall survival, patient-reported outcomes, and treatment-related complications.

RESULTS:

- The median age of participants was approximately 60 years; over 70% were male and approximately 90% had undergone prior nephrectomy. The most common sites of metastases were the lungs (78%), lymph nodes (50%), and bones (30%).
- Progression-free survival favored sunitinib by 6 months. Median progression-free survival times were 11.0 months versus 5 months in the interferon alfa group (hazard ratio [HR] 0.42; 95% confidence interval [CI], 0.32 to 0.54).
- Based on the initial interim analysis, overall survival also favored the sunitinib group (HR 0.65; 95% CI, 0.45 to 94).

- Patients in the sunitinib group reported clinically relevant improved health-related quality of life measured using the Functional Assessment of Cancer Therapy—General (FACT-G) instrument.
- Diarrhea was the most common adverse event in the sunitinib group and was much more frequent compared to the interferon alfa group (53% vs. 12%). Vomiting (24% vs. 10%) and decline in ejection fraction (10% vs. 3%) were also more common in the sunitinib group.

Criticisms and Limitations: The primary endpoint of this study was progression-free rather than overall survival, which would have been a more patient-important outcome. Generalizability is limited to patients with good performance status only and without central nervous system metastases. At the time of this study, high-dose interleukin therapy[2] was considered the most effective treatment for metastatic RCC, with complete remissions in 7% of patients. However, its use was frequently limited by severe cardiorespiratory adverse events; it nevertheless would have been a relevant comparator for this trial.

Other Relevant Studies and Information:

- In the final, unadjusted survival analyses reported secondarily, median overall survival favored the sunitinib arm (HR 0.82; 95% CI, 0.67 to 1.0) but failed to meet the predefined threshold of statistical significance. This corresponded to median overall survival times of 26.4 versus 21.8 months favoring sunitinib.[3]
- Head-to-head trials of sunitinib and pazopanib have indicated that first-line pazopanib is not inferior to sunitinib in patients with metastatic clear cell RCC[4] but may be preferred by patients due to a more favorable toxicity profile.[5]
- In a rapidly changing field, either sunitinib or pazopanib is recommended as first-line therapy in patients with treatment-naïve, favorable-risk metastatic clear cell carcinoma.[6] The combination of nivolumab and ipilimumab is favored in treatment-naïve patients of intermediate and poor risk.

Summary and Implications: This trial found sunitinib, a tyrosine kinase inhibitor, to be superior to interferon alfa for patients with metastatic RCC. Tyrosine kinase inhibitors are now among the first-line agents used in patients with metastatic RCC; other agents in this class include pazopanib, axitinib, and cabozantinib.[6]

CLINICAL CASE: FIRST-LINE TREATMENT FOR TREATMENT-NAÏVE METASTATIC RCC

Case History:

A 67-year-old male is diagnosed with metastatic clear cell RCC with multiple pulmonary metastases. He underwent a radical nephrectomy several years ago but has not had any form of systemic therapy yet. He is otherwise healthy with an excellent performance status. How should he be treated?

Suggested Answer:

This trial found that there was improved progression-free survival associated with sunitinib compared with interferon alfa, which is no longer being used, and the results appear readily applicable to him. The patient should be informed that sunitinib does not offer a curative potential, that it can have severe side effects which include gastrointestinal symptoms and fatigue, and that the gains in progression-free and potentially overall survival are relatively modest (on the order of months, not years). However, extended long-term survival is being achieved by sequencing different agents with different mechanisms of actions, such as mTOR inhibitors and immune checkpoint inhibitors.

References

1. Motzer RJ, Hutson TE, Tomczak P, et al. Sunitinib versus interferon alfa in metastatic renal-cell carcinoma. *N Engl J Med* 2007;356(2):115–24. doi: 10.1056/NEJMoa065044

2. Yang JC, Sherry RM, Steinberg SM, et al. Randomized study of high-dose and low-dose interleukin-2 in patients with metastatic renal cancer. *J Clin Oncol* 2003;21(16):3127–32. doi: 10.1200/JCO.2003.02.122 [published online first: 2003/08/14]

3. Motzer RJ, Hutson TE, Tomczak P, et al. Overall survival and updated results for sunitinib compared with interferon alfa in patients with metastatic renal cell carcinoma. *J Clin Oncol* 2009;27(22):3584–90. doi: 10.1200/JCO.2008.20.1293 [published online first: 2009/06/03]

4. Motzer RJ, Hutson TE, Cella D, et al. Pazopanib versus sunitinib in metastatic renal-cell carcinoma. *N Engl J Med* 2013;369(8):722–31. doi: 10.1056/NEJMoa1303989 [published online first: 2013/08/24]

5. Escudier B, Porta C, Bono P, et al. Randomized, controlled, double-blind, cross-over trial assessing treatment preference for pazopanib versus sunitinib in patients with metastatic renal cell carcinoma: PISCES study. *J Clin Oncol* 2014;32(14):1412–8. doi: 10.1200/JCO.2013.50.8267 [published online first: 2014/04/02]

6. Ljungberg B, Albiges L, Bensalah K, et al. Renal cell carcinoma: European Association of Urology; 2019. Available from: https://uroweb.org/guideline/renal-cell-carcinoma/?type=summary-of-changes. Accessed 1/13/2020.

22

Nivolumab Versus Everolimus in Advanced Renal Cell Carcinoma

CheckMate 025

CHRISTOPHER WEIGHT

"Among patients with previously treated advanced renal-cell carcinoma, overall survival was longer and fewer grade 3 or 4 adverse events occurred with nivolumab than with everolimus."[1]

Research Question: In patients with metastatic renal cell carcinoma (RCC) who have failed antiangiogenic therapy, how do outcomes compare with systemic therapy with nivolumab versus everolimus?

Funding: Bristol-Myers Squibb (USA)

Year Study Began: 2012

Year Study Published: 2015

Study Location: 146 sites in 24 countries in North America, Europe, Australia, South America, and Asia

Who Was Studied: Men and women over the age of 18 with metastatic clear cell RCC who had previously failed one or two antiangiogenic therapy regimens

Who Was Excluded: Patients with metastasis to the central nervous system, those who had received previous treatment with an mTOR inhibitor, and those who had a condition requiring treatment with glucocorticoids

Patients: 821

Study Overview:

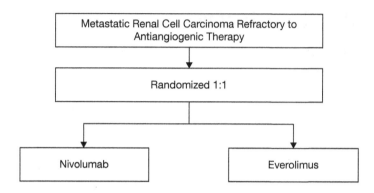

Study Interventions: Patients in the intervention arm received 3 mg nivolumab per kilogram of body weight intravenously every 2 weeks or a 10-mg everolimus tablet orally once daily. The patients were followed every 8 weeks for the first year, then every 12 weeks until disease progression or discontinuation of treatment. After discontinuation of treatment participants were allowed to start other therapies and were assessed every 3 months for survival.

Follow-up: Median 22 months

Endpoints: Primary outcome: overall survival. Secondary outcomes: objective response rate, progression-free survival, treatment-related complications, and the association between overall survival and tumor expression of PD-L1.

RESULTS:

- The mean patient age was 60 years, and approximately half the patients in both groups were intermediate risk per Memorial Sloan Kettering Cancer Center risk categories.
- Previous systemic cancer therapies were sunitinib (60%), pazopanib (30%), and axitinib (remainder).

- The median overall survival was 5.4 months longer with nivolumab, 25.0 months (95% confidence interval [CI], 21.8 to not estimable) in the nivolumab group, and 19.6 months (95% CI, 17.6 to 23.1) in the everolimus group. Hazard ratio (HR) was 0.73 (98.5% CI, 0.57 to 0.93)
- The objective response rate was higher with nivolumab than with everolimus (25% vs. 5%; odds ratio 5.98; 95% CI, 3.68 to 9.72). The median duration of response in both groups was 12 months.
- The median progression-free survival was similar between the two, 4.6 months (95% CI, 3.7 to 5.4) in the nivolumab group and 4.4 months (95% CI, 3.7 to 5.5) in the everolimus group (HR 0.88; 95% CI, 0.75 to 1.03; p = 0.11).
- Treatment-related adverse events were more common in the everolimus group than the nivolumab group. Grade 3 or 4 adverse events were noted in 37% versus 19%, respectively.
- The benefit from nivolumab treatment appeared to be irrespective of PD-L1 expression levels.

Criticism and Limitations: The trial was stopped early for benefit, which is likely to have resulted in more imprecise results and could have biased the results in favor of a larger effect size.[2] Patients previously treated with mTOR inhibitors, those with central nervous system metastasis, those with a lower performance status, and those on steroids were excluded, thereby limiting generalizability.

Other Relevant Studies and Information:

- Quality-of-life data have been separately reported, with results indicating improved quality of life with nivolumab.[3]
- CheckMate 214[4] found improved overall survival with nivolumab plus ipilimumab versus sunitinib alone among intermediate- and poor-risk patients with previously untreated advanced RCC.
- PD-1 and PD-L1 checkpoint blockade in cancer treatment is showing efficacy in many different cancer types. There are now approved drugs for lung, kidney, and bladder cancer and melanoma, with several other diseases being actively studied.[5]

Summary and Implications: This trial was the first randomized phase 3 trial for the new class of immune checkpoint blockade drugs in advanced RCC. It led to approval by the US Food and Drug Administration (FDA) of this drug for second- or third-line treatment of patients previously treated with antiangiogenic agents. This new line of potential drugs remains an area of active research, and several other checkpoint blockade drugs are under investigation in various settings of advanced RCC.

CLINICAL CASE: SECOND-LINE TREATMENT OF METASTATIC RCC

Case History:

A 59-year-old male is diagnosed with metastatic clear cell RCC. His cancer progresses on first-line therapy with axitinib, but he is otherwise healthy, with a good performance status. According to the results of this trial, what other therapeutic options does he have?

Suggested Answer:

The study found improved overall survival associated with nivolumab compared to everolimus. The described patient meets the inclusion criteria of this trial and the results should be applicable to him in his specific clinical setting. European Society of Medical Oncology (ESMO) guidelines recommend nivolumab as a standard second-line therapy in patients who have failed tyrosine kinase inhibitors,[6] and the European Association of Urology provides it with a strong recommendation after one or two lines of vascular endothelial growth factor (VEGF)-targeted therapy.[7]

References

1. Motzer RJ, Escudier B, McDermott DF, et al. Nivolumab versus everolimus in advanced renal-cell carcinoma. *N Engl J Med.* 2015;373(19):1803–13.
2. Bassler D, Briel M, Montori VM, et al. Stopping randomized trials early for benefit and estimation of treatment effects: systematic review and meta-regression analysis. *JAMA.* 2010;303(12):1180–7.
3. Cella D, Grunwald V, Nathan P, et al. Quality of life in patients with advanced renal cell carcinoma given nivolumab versus everolimus in CheckMate 025: a randomised, open-label, phase 3 trial. *Lancet Oncol.* 2016;17(7):994–1003.
4. Motzer RJ, Tannir NM, McDermott DF, et al. Nivolumab plus ipilimumab versus sunitinib in advanced renal-cell carcinoma. *N Engl J Med.* 2018;378(14):1277–90.

5. Hamanishi J, Mandai M, Matsumura N, et al. PD-1/PD-L1 blockade in cancer treatment: perspectives and issues. *Int J Clin Oncol.* 2016;21(3):462–73.

6. Escudier B, Porta C, Schmidinger M, et al. Renal cell carcinoma: ESMO clinical practice guidelines for diagnosis, treatment and follow-up. *Ann Oncol.* 2019;30(5):706–20.

7. Ljungberg B, Bensalah K, Canfield S, et al. EAU guidelines on renal cell carcinoma: 2014 update. *Eur Urol.* 2015;67(5):913–24.

23

The Effect of Intravesical Mitomycin C on Recurrence of Newly Diagnosed Superficial Bladder Cancer

A Further Report With 7 Years of Follow-Up

VIKRAM M. NARAYAN

"Our analysis confirms the positive benefit of [intravesical] mitomycin C to decrease the number of subsequent recurrences and increase the recurrence-free interval."[1]

Research Question: In patients with newly diagnosed superficial bladder cancer, does the instillation of intravesical mitomycin C (MMC) after transurethral resection prevent recurrence, recurrence rate, and disease progression?

Funding: Medical Research Council, United Kingdom

Year Study Began: 1984

Year Study Published: 1996

Study Location: 17 centers in the United Kingdom

Who Was Studied: Patients with newly diagnosed Ta or T1 transitional (urothelial) cell carcinoma of the bladder who had a World Health Organization (WHO) performance status 0 to 2

Who Was Excluded: Patients with a urinary tract infection and those with muscle-invasive bladder cancer[2]

Patients: 502

Study Overview:

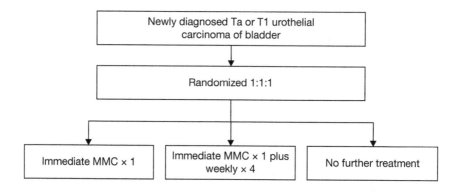

Study Intervention: Intravesical MMC (40 mg in 40 ml water) within 24 hours of transurethral resection, or intravesical MMC within 24 hours of transurethral resection plus four additional instillations within 1 year (total five instillations). Patients in the control group received no further treatment. Patients underwent cystoscopy every month for the first year, every 6 months for the second year, and annually thereafter for a total of 7 years. Patients with visual evidence for recurrence underwent biopsy.

Follow-up: Median follow-up was 7 years.

Endpoints: Primary outcomes: interval to first recurrence (recurrence-free interval) and recurrence rate during the first 2 years (number of positive cystoscopies/total follow-up interval). Secondary outcomes: progression to invasive disease, muscle metastases, death from bladder cancer (all combined to define a composite endpoint) and overall survival.

RESULTS:

- 5-year recurrence-free rate was 40% in the control group, 55% in group 1 (single instillation of MMC), and 63% in group 2 (five instillations of mitomycin C).
- Compared to controls, both MMC groups had reduced rates of subsequent recurrences (34% for group 1, p = 0.01; 50% for group 2, p = 0.0001).
- Although comparing groups 1 and 2 seemed to suggest a benefit with additional instillations, no benefit was proven (p = 0.10).
- Progression-free interval was not different among the three groups.
- There was no difference in overall survival among the three groups.
- Toxicity/side effects were minimal, though the authors note that delayed healing at the resection site was observed in a few cases.

Criticisms and Limitations: Nearly 10% of patients randomized were excluded from the analysis, which highlights the real-world challenge in selecting patients for this therapy based on the urologist's visual assessment of whether the tumor is superficial and/or low grade. Up to a third of participants in trials of intravesical agents may have been excluded from analyses due to a pathologic finding of either muscle-invasive tumor or no malignancy at all.[3] At the time of an interim analysis after a median follow-up of 12 months, follow-up was available for only 397 of 502 patients,[2] whereas rates of follow-up at the time of final analysis are unclear,[4] raising concerns about attrition bias.

Other Relevant Studies and Information:

- A systematic review and individual patient data meta-analysis of randomized controlled trials comparing a single immediate instillation of chemotherapy after transurethral resection to resection alone found that instillation reduces the risk of recurrence by 35% (hazard ratio 0.65; 95% confidence interval, 0.58 to 0.74, p < 0.001); however, this benefit was not seen in patients at high risk for recurrence.[4]
- Guidelines from both the American Urological Association (AUA)[5] and the European Association of Urology (EAU)[6] for non-muscle-invasive bladder cancer recommend a single immediate instillation of intravesical chemotherapy in patients with small-volume, low-grade Ta tumors.

- Mitomycin is also used for additional adjuvant intravesical chemotherapy instillations; however, bacillus Calmette–Guérin (BCG) induction and maintenance therapy is probably superior in reducing the risk of recurrence.[7]
- A single intravesical instillation of MMC may also reduce the risk of urothelial carcinoma recurrence after nephroureterectomy for upper tract urothelial carcinoma.[8]

Summary and Implications: This study was the first to demonstrate that a single immediate instillation of MMC following transurethral resection of a suspected noninvasive urothelial cell carcinoma confers a reduced risk of disease recurrence.

CLINICAL CASE: SINGLE-DOSE INTRAVESICAL MMC ADMINISTRATION AFTER TRANSURETHRAL BLADDER CANCER RESECTION

Case History:

A 45-year-old male presents with gross hematuria. He undergoes a diagnostic cystoscopy, which reveals two 1-cm papillary-type lesions emanating from the right lateral wall. How should he be counseled?

Suggested Answer:

This patient has what appears to be low-grade bladder cancer, although at this point the diagnosis is not histologically confirmed. He should be offered a transurethral resection with a single dose of MMC instilled intravesically after the procedure, assuming the surgeon has no suspicions after resection of bladder injury or invasive disease. According to the Tolley et al. study,[1,2] intravesical MMC, if administered either as a single dose postoperatively or along with four additional instillations over the course of a year, will reduce the rate of disease recurrence. Current EAU and AUA guidelines recommend a single postoperative dose, which should be administered within 24 hours of transurethral resection.[5,6] If there is any overt or suspected bladder perforation, this should be omitted.

References

1. Tolley DA, Parmar MK, Grigor KM, et al. The effect of intravesical mitomycin C on recurrence of newly diagnosed superficial bladder cancer: a further report with 7 years of follow-up. *J Urol* 1996;155(4):1233–8.

2. Tolley DA, Hargreave TB, Smith PH, et al. Effect of intravesical mitomycin C on recurrence of newly diagnosed superficial bladder cancer: interim report from the Medical Research Council Subgroup on Superficial Bladder Cancer (Urological Cancer Working Party). *Br Med J (Clin Res Ed)* 1988;296(6639):1759–61. doi: 10.1136/bmj.296.6639.1759 [published online first: 1988/06/25]

3. Holmang S. Early single-instillation chemotherapy has no real benefit and should be abandoned in non-muscle-invasive bladder cancer. *Eur Urol Suppl* 2009;8(5):458–63. doi: doi:10.1016/j.eursup.2008.12.003

4. Malmstrom PU, Sylvester RJ, Crawford DE, et al. An individual patient data meta-analysis of the long-term outcome of randomised studies comparing intravesical mitomycin C versus bacillus Calmette-Guerin for non-muscle-invasive bladder cancer. *Eur Urol* 2009;56(2):247–56. doi: 10.1016/j.eururo.2009.04.038 [published online first: 2009/05/05]

5. Chang SS, Bochner BH, Chou R, et al. Treatment of non-metastatic muscle-invasive bladder cancer: AUA/ASCO/ASTRO/SUO guideline. *J Urol* 2017;198(3):552–59. doi: 10.1016/j.juro.2017.04.086 [published online first: 2017/05/01]

6. Babjuk M, Burger M, Comperat EM, et al. European Association of Urology guidelines on non-muscle-invasive bladder cancer (TaT1 and carcinoma in situ)— 2019 update. *Eur Urol* 2019;76(5):639–57. doi: 10.1016/j.eururo.2019.08.016 [published online first: 2019/08/25]

7. Schmidt S, Kunath F, Coles B, et al. Intravesical bacillus Calmette-Guerin versus mitomycin C for Ta and T1 bladder cancer. *Cochrane Database Syst Rev* 2020;1:CD011935. doi: 10.1002/14651858.CD011935.pub2 [published online first: 2020/01/09]

8. Hwang EC, Sathianathen NJ, Jung JH, et al. Single-dose intravesical chemotherapy after nephroureterectomy for upper tract urothelial carcinoma. *Cochrane Database Syst Rev* 2019;5:CD013160. doi: 10.1002/14651858.CD013160.pub2 [published online first: 2019/05/19]

24

Bacillus Calmette–Guérin (BCG) Immunotherapy for Recurrent Noninvasive Transitional Cell Carcinoma of the Bladder

A Randomized Southwest Oncology Group (SWOG) Study

VIKRAM M. NARAYAN

> "Compared to standard induction therapy maintenance BCG immunotherapy was beneficial in patients with carcinoma in situ and select patients with Ta, T1 bladder cancer. Median recurrence-free survival time was twice as long in the 3-week maintenance arm compared to the no maintenance arm, and patients had significantly longer worsening-free survival."[1]

Research Question: Does maintenance intravesical BCG reduce the risk for recurrence or progression of high-grade superficial or carcinoma in situ (CIS) transitional cell carcinoma?

Funding: National Cancer Institute

Year Study Began: 1985

Year Study Published: 2000

Study Location: 81 SWOG locations

Who Was Studied: Patients with completely resected stage Ta (noninvasive urothelial confined) or T1 (lamina propria invasion) urothelial cell carcinoma, with an increased risk of recurrence (defined as two tumors within 1 year, three or more within the most recent 6 months, and/or CIS on at least one random biopsy). Patients who had received intravesical chemotherapy were eligible.

Who Was Excluded: Patients with muscle-invasive disease and those who has previously received BCG treatment.

Patients: 550

Study Overview:

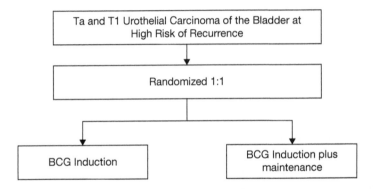

Study Intervention: All patients were given induction therapy 1 week after tumor resection, which comprised six weekly treatments of intravesical (81 mg of Connaught BCG suspended in 50 cc saline) and percutaneous BCG. Intravesical BCG was administered through a urethral catheter and patients were requested to retain it for 2 hours, while percutaneous BCG was administered to the inner thigh.

Following induction, patients without evidence of disease recurrence were randomized into either the maintenance-therapy or no-maintenance-therapy arm. Maintenance therapy comprised three successive weekly intravesical and percutaneous administrations of BCG at 3 months, 6 months, and every 6 months thereafter to 3 years from the start of induction therapy. Patients with CIS underwent bladder biopsy at 3 and 6 months, and thereafter if indicated by suspicious urine cytology or cystoscopy.

Follow-Up: Median follow-up was not explicitly provided.

Endpoints: Primary outcome: recurrence-free survival, and in patients with CIS, histological disappearance of malignancy on bladder biopsy and resolution of abnormal cytology. Secondary outcomes: disease progression (biopsy evidence of stage T2 or higher, need for cystectomy, systemic chemotherapy, radiation, or other therapy indicating abandonment of treatment of superficial disease alone).

RESULTS:

- Patient mean age was 67 years; approximately one-third had CIS.
- Recurrence-free survival rates at 5 years were 60% and 41% in the maintenance and no-maintenance arms, respectively; median times were 76.8 (64.3 to 93.2) and 35.7 (25.1 to 56.8) months, respectively.
- Disease progression-free survival rates at 5 years were 76% and 70%, also favoring the maintenance arm, whereas overall survival rates were similar.
- 2 of 599 patients died due to septic complications at the time of induction. No grade 3 or higher toxicities were reported in the maintenance arm.
- Only 16% of patients in the maintenance arm received all eight scheduled treatments over 3 years.

Criticisms and Limitations: Outcome analyses were based on only 284 of 550 randomized patients (51.6%), raising major concerns over attrition bias. There is no indication that patients, personnel, or outcome assessors were blinded, raising concerns over performance and detection bias. Although few adverse events were reported, few study participants completed all scheduled treatments, underscoring the high burden of treatment-related side effects and the real-world challenges in promoting adherence to maintenance schedules.

Other Relevant Studies and Information:

- The administration of percutaneous BCG in the study protocol reflects the original description of BCG immunotherapy for bladder cancer by Morales et al.[2] Other studies have since demonstrated similar outcomes with intravesical BCG alone, and percutaneous BCG administration has since been abandoned.[3]

- Published studies vary in the type of BCG strain administered, with the most common ones being Tice, Connaught, Pasteur, RIVM, and A. Frappier.
- A meta-analysis of four trials involving 645 patients evaluating the use of maintenance BCG found that the therapy reduced recurrence rates by 14% (95% confidence interval, –26 to –1) when compared to induction therapy alone.[5,6]
- Current European Association of Urology guidelines recommend BCG induction and maintenance treatment for 3 years.[4] The American Urological Association recommends these in both intermediate- and high-risk patients.[5]

Summary and Implications: This study was the first to suggest that maintenance BCG reduces disease-specific recurrence in noninvasive bladder cancers. It may also reduce the rate of disease progression to T2 or greater, but this has been drawn into question.[6] The recommended maintenance regimen is a 6-week induction course of BCG after transurethral resection, followed by 3-week maintenance instillations at 3 and 6 months, followed by every 6 months thereafter up to 36 months. Many patients do not tolerate the full SWOG maintenance regimen due to treatment-related side effects, most commonly symptoms of cystitis and hematuria, as well as rarely high-grade fever and BCG sepsis.

CLINICAL CASE: BCG MAINTENANCE THERAPY FOR UROTHELIAL BLADDER CANCER

Case History:
A 64-year-old woman is newly diagnosed with high-grade noninvasive urothelial cell carcinoma, found after transurethral resection of two separate lesions in the bladder. How should she be counseled?

Suggested Answer:
Based on current guidelines, she should undergo re-resection to rule out muscle-invasive disease.[4,5] Assuming she does not have contraindications to therapy (immunosuppression, personal history of BCG sepsis, gross hematuria, recent traumatic catheterization, severe liver disease, or total incontinence precluding her ability to retain the agent), this patient should be offered a 6-week course of induction BCG after recovering from her resection, followed by maintenance BCG according to the SWOG regimen. She should be appropriately counseled on the risks of BCG toxicity, including severe irritative lower urinary tract symptoms, allergic reactions, and BCG sepsis.

References

1. Lamm DL, Blumenstein BA, Crissman JD, et al. Maintenance bacillus Calmette-Guerin immunotherapy for recurrent TA, T1 and carcinoma in situ transitional cell carcinoma of the bladder: a randomized Southwest Oncology Group Study. *J Urol* 2000;163(4):1124–9.

2. Morales A, Eidinger D, Bruce AW. Intracavitary bacillus Calmette-Guerin in the treatment of superficial bladder tumors. *J Urol* 1976;116(2):180–3. doi: 10.1016/s0022-5347(17)58737-6 [published online first: 1976/08/01]

3. Badalament RA, Herr HW, Wong GY, et al. A prospective randomized trial of maintenance versus nonmaintenance intravesical bacillus Calmette-Guerin therapy of superficial bladder cancer. *J Clin Oncol* 1987;5(3):441–9. doi: 10.1200/JCO.1987.5.3.441 [published online first: 1987/03/01]

4. Babjuk M, Burger M, Comperat EM, et al. European Association of Urology guidelines on non-muscle-invasive bladder cancer (TaT1 and carcinoma in situ)—2019 update. *Eur Urol* 2019;76(5):639–57. doi: 10.1016/j.eururo.2019.08.016 [published online first: 2019/08/25]

5. Chang SS, Bochner BH, Chou R, et al. Treatment of non-metastatic muscle-invasive bladder cancer: AUA/ASCO/ASTRO/SUO guideline. *J Urol* 2017;198(3):552–9. doi: 10.1016/j.juro.2017.04.086 [published online first: 2017/05/01]

6. Sylvester RJ, van der MA, Lamm DL. Intravesical bacillus Calmette-Guerin reduces the risk of progression in patients with superficial bladder cancer: a meta-analysis of the published results of randomized clinical trials. *J Urol* 2002;168(5):1964–70. doi: 10.1097/01.ju.0000034450.80198.1c [published online first: 2002/10/24]

25

Neoadjuvant Chemotherapy Plus Cystectomy Compared With Cystectomy Alone for Locally Advanced Bladder Cancer

VIKRAM M. NARAYAN

"As compared with radical cystectomy alone, the use of neoadjuvant methotrexate, vinblastine, doxorubicin, and cisplatin followed by radical cystectomy . . . is associated with improved survival among patients with locally advanced bladder cancer."[1]

Research Question: Does neoadjuvant methotrexate, vinblastine, doxorubicin, and cisplatin (M-VAC) improve the survival of patients with locally advanced bladder cancer?

Funding: US National Cancer Institute and US Department of Health and Human Services

Year Study Began: 1987

Year Study Published: 2003

Study Location: 126 institutions affiliated with the Southwest Oncology Group, Eastern
   Cooperative Oncology Group, or Cancer and Leukemia Group B

Who Was Studied: Radical cystectomy candidates with stage T2N0M0 to T4aN0M0 bladder cancer who had adequate renal, hepatic, and hematologic function; who had a Karnofsky performance status of 0 or 1; and who had not undergone radiation

Patients: 317

Study Overview:

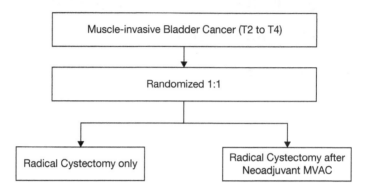

- Randomized controlled trial with stratification based on age (younger than 65 years vs. 65 years or older) and stage (T2 vs. T3 or T4a)
- Patients were randomly allocated to undergo radical cystectomy alone or to receive three cycles of M-VAC chemotherapy prior to radical cystectomy; radical cystectomy included a bilateral pelvic lymphadenectomy. Urinary diversion type (i.e., ileal conduit or neobladder) varied.
- Biopsies of tumor were obtained prior to trial registration, and cystectomy specimens were reviewed after surgery to assess pathologic downstaging, if present.

Study Intervention: Patients in the intervention group received three cycles (28 days) of M-VAC prior to radical cystectomy. Those in the control group received a standard radical cystectomy.

Follow-Up: Median follow-up was 8.7 years (MVAC + cystectomy group) and 8.4 years (cystectomy-alone group).

Endpoints: Primary outcome: overall survival. Secondary outcome: tumor stage at the time of radical cystectomy (as the result of downstaging).

RESULTS:

- 82% of the patients randomized to combination therapy underwent cystectomy as planned, compared to 81% of those in the cystectomy-alone group.
- In an intention-to-treat analysis, at 5 years, 57% of patients in the combination-therapy group were alive, compared to 43% of those in the cystectomy-only group. However, these results did not reach statistical significance ($p = 0.06$).
- Median overall survival time in the combination therapy group was 77 months, compared to 46 months for patients who underwent cystectomy alone ($p = 0.05$).
- Significant disease downstaging was noted in the combination-therapy arm, with 38% of surgical specimens from these patients achieving pT0 status (pathologically free of cancer) at the time of surgery, compared to only 15% being pT0 in the cystectomy-alone arm ($p < 0.001$).
- No deaths were attributed to M-VAC therapy and there were no differences between the two groups with respect to the severity of postoperative complications. Among patients who underwent chemotherapy, 33% had severe granulocytopenia, while 17% had moderate gastrointestinal symptoms.

Criticisms and Limitations:

- The survival analysis did not reach statistical significance, even when stratified by age (greater than 65 years vs. less than 65 years) or tumor stage (T2 vs. T3 or greater). This is consistent with other trials of neoadjuvant chemotherapy and may reflect issues with respect to sample size and early study closure.
- The authors did not specify the frequency of follow-up. It is therefore possible that those who underwent combination therapy were followed more closely (given the additional monitoring necessitated by the need for following chemotherapy-related adverse effects), potentially conferring a survival advantage due to prompter recognition of disease recurrence.

Other Relevant Studies and Information:

- The Advanced Bladder Cancer Meta-analysis Collaboration in 2005 performed a systematic review and meta-analysis of individual patient data from 11 randomized controlled trials, including this study. Platinum-based combination neoadjuvant chemotherapy was associated with a significant survival benefit (hazard ratio [HR] 0.86; 95% confidence interval [CI], 0.77 to 0.95; p = 0.003), equivalent to a 5% absolute improvement in survival at 5 years. The meta-analysis also demonstrated a significant disease-free survival benefit at 5 years (HR 0.78; 95% CI, 0.71 to 0.86; p < 0.0001).[1]

- The European Association of Urology guidelines currently recommend cisplatin-based neoadjuvant chemotherapy for patients with clinical T2-T4aN0M0 bladder cancer.[2]
- The National Comprehensive Cancer Network (NCCN) guidelines recommend strong consideration of neoadjuvant cisplatin-based chemotherapy for cT2N0M0 patients and recommend it for cT3-T4aN0M0 patients.[3]
- Neoadjuvant chemotherapy for bladder cancer has historically been underutilized in the United States, with only 1.4% and 11% of cT2 and cT4 patients receiving it between 1992 and 2002, based on Surveillance, Epidemiology, and End Results (SEER) Medicare data.[4] There has been recent improvement, with a study showing that neoadjuvant chemotherapy was used in 29.5% of cases in 2006 and 39.8% of cases in 2010 (p < 0.001).[5]

Summary and Implications: In combination with a subsequent systematic review and individual patient meta-analysis, this trial suggests that neoadjuvant chemotherapy confers a benefit with regard to overall survival among patients with locally advanced bladder cancer. Platinum-based combination chemotherapy also confers disease downstaging in patients with cT2-T4a nonmetastatic bladder cancer prior to radical cystectomy, without an apparent increase in the complication rate after surgery.. Eligible patients (i.e., those with T2-T4aN0M0) should be offered neoadjuvant chemotherapy prior to radical cystectomy, though poor performance status and impaired renal function remain barriers to more widespread use.

CLINICAL CASE: LOCALLY ADVANCED BLADDER CANCER

Case History:

A 63-year-old male is found to have a 5-cm mass at the bladder dome. Transurethral resection reveals urothelial cell carcinoma invading the muscularis propria. A staging computed tomography scan of the chest, abdomen, and pelvis shows no evidence for metastatic disease. Based on the results of this trial, what treatment do you recommend for this patient?

Suggested Answer:

The SWOG trial found that providing patients with three cycles of M-VAC chemotherapy prior to radical cystectomy conferred an improved median survival over patients who received chemotherapy alone (77 vs. 46 months). Moreover, significant disease downstaging was noted in the combination-therapy arm, with nearly 38% of patients (compared to 15% among those who did not receive chemotherapy) achieving pT0 status at the time of surgery. Absence of residual cancer in the cystectomy specimen was associated with improved survival. It is not clear whether this patient would be a good candidate for chemotherapy, however, given the absence of information on performance status and his baseline renal function, both of which need to be evaluated and remain an ongoing barrier to widespread utilization of neoadjuvant chemotherapy in the United States.

References

1. Advanced Bladder Cancer Meta-Analysis Collaboration. Neoadjuvant chemotherapy in invasive bladder cancer: update of a systematic review and meta-analysis of individual patient data advanced bladder cancer (ABC) meta-analysis collaboration. *Eur Urol.* 2005;48:202–256. doi:10.1016/j.eururo.2005.04.006.
2. Witjes JA, Compérat E, Cowan NC, et al. EAU guidelines on muscle-invasive and metastatic bladder cancer: summary of the 2013 guidelines. *Eur Urol.* 2014;65(4):778–792. doi:10.1016/j.eururo.2013.11.046.
3. Clark PE, Spiess PE, Agarwal N, et al. NCCN clinical practice guidelines in oncology (NCCN Guidelines®): bladder cancer. *Natl Compr Cancer Netw.* 2016;14(10):1213–1224. doi:10.6004/jnccn.2016.0131.
4. Porter MP, Kerrigan MC, Donato BMK, Ramsey SD. Patterns of use of systemic chemotherapy for Medicare beneficiaries with urothelial bladder cancer. *Urol Oncol Semin Orig Investig.* 2011;29(3):252–258. doi:10.1016/j.urolonc.2009.03.021.
5. Reardon ZD, Patel SG, Zaid HB, et al. Trends in the use of perioperative chemotherapy for localized and locally advanced muscle-invasive bladder cancer: a sign of changing tides. *Eur Urol.* 2015;67(1):165–170. doi:10.1016/j.eururo.2014.01.009.

26

Radiotherapy With or Without Chemotherapy in Muscle-Invasive Bladder Cancer

VIKRAM M. NARAYAN

"[O]ur study shows that the addition of chemotherapy to radiotherapy improved local control, particularly freedom from invasive recurrence, as compared with radiotherapy alone, and resulted in good long-term bladder function and low rates of salvage cystectomy, all of which are of major importance in this elderly, relatively frail group of patients."[1]

Research Question: In patients with nonmetastatic invasive bladder cancer, how does local radiotherapy compare with or without radiosensitizing chemotherapy?

Funding: Cancer Research UK and the National Institute for Health Research

Year Study Began: 2001

Year Study Published: 2012

Study Location: 45 centers in the United Kingdom

Who Was Studied: Patients over the age of 18 with histologically confirmed T2, T3, or T4a N0M0 disease with a performance status of 0 to 2

Who Was Excluded: Patients who were pregnant, patients who previously had cancer or radiotherapy, or patients with inflammatory bowel disease

Patients: 360

Study Overview:

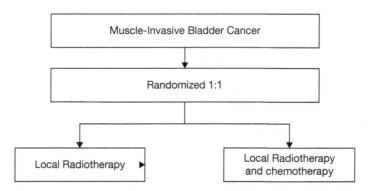

Study Intervention: Patients were randomized to undergo radiotherapy with or without synchronous chemotherapy with intravenous 5-fluorouracil (500 mg/m^2 per 24 hours on weeks 1 and 4 of treatment) and intravenous mitomycin (12 mg/m^2) on day 1. A second (optional participation) randomization took place for whole-bladder radiotherapy or modified volume randomization. Centers could opt to administer either 55 Gy in 20 fractions over 4 weeks or 64 Gy in 32 fractions over 6.5 weeks, with dose modifications for both chemotherapy and radiotherapy permitted. The initial accrual goal was 460 patients; this was reduced to 350 patients due to poor accrual, accepting a reduced statistical power. Patients were followed weekly during treatment. Following conclusion of treatment they were seen at 6 months and 9 months after randomization and annually thereafter.

Follow-Up: Median follow-up was approximately 70 months.

Endpoints: Primary outcome: locoregional (pelvic) disease-free survival. Secondary outcomes: late toxicity at 1 and 2 years, bladder capacity, and quality of life. Additional measures included acute toxicity; local control per cystoscopy at 3, 12, and 24 months; rate of salvage cystectomy; and overall survival.

RESULTS:

- The 2-year locoregional recurrence-free survival rates were 67% (95% confidence interval [CI], 59 to 74) in the chemoradiotherapy group and 54% (95% CI, 46 to 62) in the radiotherapy group, translating to a

hazard ratio of 0.68 favoring chemoradiotherapy (95% CI, 0.48 to 0.96; p = 0.03).
- Relapses included:
  - Invasive bladder cancer in 20 patients (11.0%) in the chemoradiotherapy group and 34 patients (19.1%) in the radiotherapy group
  - Non-muscle-invasive bladder cancer in 26 patients (14.3%) in the chemoradiotherapy group and 30 (16.9%) in the radiotherapy group
  - Pelvic node relapse in 9 patients (4.9%) in the chemoradiotherapy group and 12 (6.7%) in the radiotherapy group
- 5-year overall survival rates were 48% (95% CI, 40 to 55) in the chemoradiotherapy group versus 35% (95% CI, 28 to 43) in the radiotherapy group for a hazard ratio of 0.82 (95% CI, 0.63 to 1.09). There were 208 deaths, 98 in the chemoradiotherapy group and 110 in the radiotherapy group.
- 51 patients underwent cystectomy as secondary treatment; rates were 11.4% in the chemoradiotherapy group compared to 16.8% on the radiotherapy group (p = 0.07). Grade 3 or 4 toxic events (primarily gastrointestinal) occurred in 36% of the chemoradiotherapy group, compared with 27.5% in the radiotherapy group, for a calculated risk ratio of 1.3 (95% CI, 1.0 to 1.3).

Criticisms and Limitations: The primary endpoint of this study was locoregional disease-free survival, and data were censored at the first sign of metastasis, despite metastatic disease remaining a significant contributor to bladder cancer morbidity and mortality. The study was underpowered to meet its original objectives, which may have contributed to the inconclusive results in terms of overall survival.

Other Relevant Studies and Information:

- Previously published data had been limited to retrospective series/convenience cohorts, with one study having demonstrated 5- and 10-year overall survival rates of 40% and 19%, respectively, with response rates dependent on disease stage.[2]
- Current evidence-based guidelines by the European Association of Urology reserve radiotherapy for patients with muscle-invasive bladder cancer who are unfit or unwilling to undergo radical cystectomy and

urinary diversion. In those patients, combination with a radiosensitizer such as cisplatin, 5-fluorouracil/mitomycin C, carbogen/nicotinamide, or gemcitabine is recommended.[3]

Summary and Implications: This study represented the first randomized controlled trial evaluating the use of radiotherapy and chemoradiotherapy for the management of invasive bladder cancer. Chemoradiotherapy with fluorouracil and mitomycin C improves locoregional disease-free survival at 2 years compared to radiotherapy alone, but there was no demonstrated impact on all-cause 5-year survival, disease-specific survival, or disease-free survival. Use of chemoradiotherapy for the treatment of invasive bladder cancer may be beneficial in well-selected patients who are otherwise poor candidates for definitive surgery and neoadjuvant chemotherapy.

CLINICAL CASE: BLADDER-PRESERVING MULTIMODALITY THERAPY FOR MUSCLE-INVASIVE BLADDER CANCER

Case History:

A 77-year-old male with severe congestive heart failure, peripheral vascular disease, and chronic obstructive pulmonary disease (COPD) on home oxygen is diagnosed with T2 urothelial cell carcinoma of the bladder. He has dyspnea with moderate exertion and hypertension. He is a prior 50-pack-year smoker, having quit 10 years ago. His baseline serum creatinine is 2.4 mg/dl. What treatment options could be considered?

Suggested Answer:

The gold standard for management of invasive bladder cancer is radical cystectomy with platinum-based neoadjuvant chemotherapy. In this patient with numerous comorbidities and poor renal function, the American College of Surgeons' NSQIP surgical risk calculator estimates his risk of serious complications at 41% and death at 5.1%, both of which are above the national average for those undergoing this procedure.[4] The trial by James et al.[1] provides evidence suggesting that improved locoregional disease-free survival may be conferred with chemoradiotherapy (5-fluorouracil and mitomycin) compared to radiotherapy alone. Chemoradiotherapy may be an option offered to this patient, with the stipulation that these data do not compare the intervention to definitive surgery and it was tested primarily among a healthier cohort of patients. Alternative treatment options include radical transurethral resection or a partial cystectomy, although both carry surgical risks.

References

1. James ND, Hussain SA, Hall E, et al. Radiotherapy with or without chemotherapy in muscle-invasive bladder cancer. *N Engl J Med* 2012;366(16):1477–88. doi: 10.1056/ NEJMoa1106106

2. Rodel C, Grabenbauer GG, Kuhn R, et al. Combined-modality treatment and selective organ preservation in invasive bladder cancer: long-term results. *J Clin Oncol* 2002;20(14):3061–71. doi: 10.1200/JCO.2002.11.027 [published online first: 2002/07/16]

3. Witjes JA, Bruins HM, Cathomas R, et al. European Association of Urology guideline on muscle-invasive and metastatic bladder cancer 2020. Available from: https:// uroweb.org/guideline/bladder-cancer-muscle-invasive-and-metastatic/#7. Accessed 2/25/2020.

4. Bilimoria KY, Liu Y, Paruch JL, et al. Development and evaluation of the universal ACS NSQIP surgical risk calculator: a decision aid and informed consent tool for patients and surgeons. *J Am Coll Surg* 2013;217(5):833–42. doi: 10.1016/ j.jamcollsurg.2013.07.385 [published online first: 2013/09/24]

27

A Randomized Comparison of Cisplatin Alone or in Combination With Methotrexate, Vinblastine, and Doxorubicin in Patients With Metastatic Urothelial Carcinoma

A Cooperative Group Study

PHILIPP DAHM AND VIKRAM M. NARAYAN

"Although a more toxic regimen, we found M-VAC to be superior to single-agent cisplatin with respect to response rate, duration of remission, and overall survival in patients with advanced urothelial carcinoma"[1]

Research Question: In patients with advanced urothelial carcinoma of the bladder, how does the addition of methotrexate, vinblastine, and doxorubicin to cisplatin (M-VAC) compare to cisplatin alone?

Funding: National Cancer Institute of Canada, US National Cancer Institute, and the Australian Public Health Service

Year Study Began: 1994

Year Study Published: 1992

Study Location: Patients from tertiary care centers in the United States, Canada, and Australia

Who Was Studied: Patients with advanced urothelial cell carcinoma of the bladder or upper tract. Eligible patients needed to have bidimensionally measurable metastases not within a field of previous radiation therapy, to have a Karnofsky performance score of 60% or more, to have recovered from previous major surgery, and to be at least 4 weeks beyond prior radiotherapy.

Who Was Excluded: Patients without adequate renal function (creatinine clearance less than 60 ml/min) and those with prior systemic therapy, history of prior malignancy, an unresolved bacterial infection, or severe cardiovascular disease

Patients: 269

Study Overview:

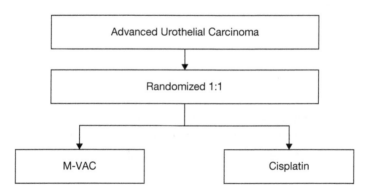

Study Interventions: Patients in the control arm received cisplatin alone (70 mg/m^2) administered intravenously on day 1 or combination chemotherapy consisting of methotrexate (30 mg/m^2) on days 1, 15, and 22; vinblastine (3 mg/m^2) on day 2; doxorubicin (30 mg/m^2) on day 2; and cisplatin (70 mg/m^2) on day 2. Courses were repeated every 28 days. Doses were adjusted or held for adverse effects or lab alterations.

Follow-up: 19.7 months (for patients still alive)

Endpoints: Primary outcome: not defined. Other outcomes: overall survival, progression-free survival, and adverse effects.

RESULTS:

- Patient median age was approximately 65 years and 80% of participants were male.
- Approximately 70% of patients had a Karnofsky performance status of 80% or greater.
- Median survival times for patients treated with the combination regimen were 12.5 months for M-VAC and 8.2 months for single-agent cisplatin $(p = 0.0002)$.
- The median progression-free survival was 10 months with M-VAC and 4.3 months for cisplatin alone (no p-value provided); overall response rates were 39.0% and 11.6%, respectively.
- There were five (4%) drug-related deaths in the M-VAC group and none (0%) in the single-agent cisplatin group $(p = 0.21)$.
- There were eight events of sepsis in the M-VAC arm compared to none in the cisplatin arm; grade 3 or 4 mucositis (17% vs. 0%) and nausea and vomiting (12% vs. 1%) were much more common in the M-VAC arm.

Criticism and Limitations: The study provides no information as to whether the assessors of response rates and progression-free survival were blinded or not. The study did not assess health-related quality of life. Applicability of the study findings is limited to patients with normal or near-normal renal function and a good performance status.

Other Relevant Studies and Information:

- A prior single-armed study of M-VAC had demonstrated high response rates with objective remissions in more than 70% of treated patients with a median survival of 13 months and provided the impetus for this trial.[2]
- Subsequent trials have since also demonstrated the effectiveness of M-VAC in the neoadjuvant and adjuvant setting.[3,4]
- M-VAC is better tolerated when combined with granulocyte colony-stimulating factor (G-CSF)[5], and high-dose intensity MVAC (HD-MVAC) combined with G-CSF may be less toxic and may have improved 2-year survival rates.[6] Long-term survival rates appear to be similar, though.[7]
- Chemotherapy with gemcitabine and cisplatin (GC) has since been demonstrated to provide a similar survival benefit compared to M-VAC

with an improved safety and side-effect profile[8] and is less nephrotoxic; at many centers it has replaced standard-of-care for treatment of advanced urothelial cell carcinoma.

Summary and Implications: This study found cisplatin-based combination therapy using the M-VAC regimen to be more effective than cisplatin alone in patients with advanced urothelial cell carcinoma, and it was able to achieve median survival times of over a year.[9] However, the regimen is associated with substantial treatment-related toxicity, including sepsis and treatment-related death.

CLINICAL CASE: CHEMOTHERAPY FOR ADVANCED UROTHELIAL CARCINOMA

Case History:

A 75-year-old male with an 80-pack-year history of tobacco abuse, chronic obstructive pulmonary disease, and peripheral vascular disease is diagnosed with muscle-invasive urothelial carcinoma of the bladder. Staging studies raise concerns about enlarged pelvic lymph nodes as well as multiple pulmonary nodules. One of the pulmonary lesions is biopsied and confirmed to be metastatic urothelial carcinoma. How should the patient be counseled?

Suggested Answer:

This patient has urothelial carcinoma that has spread beyond the bladder. His prognosis will likely be determined by his metastatic spread rather than his locoregional disease. Rather than undergoing radical cystectomy and urinary diversion, the patient should be referred to a medical oncologist for consideration of systemic chemotherapy. Based on current European Association of Urology guidelines, he would be recommended to undergo cisplatin-based chemotherapy as first-line treatment either in the form of GC or M-VAC, the latter ideally as HD-MVAC combined with G-CSF.[9] His ability to receive M-VAC chemotherapy will hinge on his performance status as well as renal and hepatic function. A discussion of serious potential side effects of this regimen needs to be part of the shared decision-making process.

References

1. Loehrer PJ, Sr., Einhorn LH, Elson PJ, et al. A randomized comparison of cisplatin alone or in combination with methotrexate, vinblastine, and doxorubicin in patients with metastatic urothelial carcinoma: a cooperative group study. *J Clin*

Oncol 1992;10(7):1066–73. doi: 10.1200/JCO.1992.10.7.1066 [published online first: 1992/07/11]

2. Sternberg CN, Yagoda A, Scher HI, et al. Methotrexate, vinblastine, doxorubicin, and cisplatin for advanced transitional cell carcinoma of the urothelium: efficacy and patterns of response and relapse. *Cancer* 1989;64(12):2448–58.

3. Advanced Bladder Cancer (ABC) Meta-analysis Collaboration. Adjuvant chemotherapy in invasive bladder cancer: a systematic review and meta-analysis of individual patient data. *Eur Urol* 2005;48(2):189–99; discussion 199–201. doi: 10.1016/j.eururo.2005.04.005

4. Vale CL. Adjuvant chemotherapy for invasive bladder cancer (individual patient data). *Cochrane Database of Systematic Reviews* 2006;(2):CD006018. doi: 10.1002/14651858.CD006018

5. Gabrilove JL, Jakubowski A, Scher H, et al. Effect of granulocyte colony-stimulating factor on neutropenia and associated morbidity due to chemotherapy for transitional-cell carcinoma of the urothelium. *N Engl J Med* 1988;318(22):1414–22. doi: 10.1056/NEJM198806023182202 [published online first: 1988/06/02]

6. Sternberg CN, de Mulder PH, Schornagel JH, et al. Randomized phase III trial of high-dose-intensity methotrexate, vinblastine, doxorubicin, and cisplatin (MVAC) chemotherapy and recombinant human granulocyte colony-stimulating factor versus classic MVAC in advanced urothelial tract tumors: European Organization for Research and Treatment of Cancer Protocol no. 30924. *J Clin Oncol* 2001;19(10):2638–46. doi: 10.1200/JCO.2001.19.10.2638 [published online first: 2001/05/16]

7. Sternberg CN, de Mulder P, Schornagel JH, et al. Seven-year update of an EORTC phase III trial of high-dose intensity M-VAC chemotherapy and G-CSF versus classic M-VAC in advanced urothelial tract tumours. *Eur J Cancer* 2006;42(1):50–4. doi: 10.1016/j.ejca.2005.08.032 [published online first: 2005/12/07]

8. von der Maase H, Hansen SW, Roberts JT, et al. Gemcitabine and cisplatin versus methotrexate, vinblastine, doxorubicin, and cisplatin in advanced or metastatic bladder cancer: results of a large, randomized, multinational, multicenter, phase III study. *J Clin Oncol* 2000;18(17):3068–77. doi: 10.1200/JCO.2000.18.17.3068 [published online first: 2000/09/23]

9. Witjes JA, Bruins HM, Cathomas R, et al. European Association of Urology guideline on muscle-invasive and metastatic bladder cancer 2020. Available from: https://uroweb.org/guideline/bladder-cancer-muscle-invasive-and-metastatic/#7. Accessed 2/25/2020.

28

Gemcitabine and Cisplatin Versus Methotrexate, Vinblastine, Doxorubicin, and Cisplatin in Advanced or Metastatic Bladder Cancer

Results of a Large, Randomized, Multinational, Multicenter, Phase III Study

VIKRAM M. NARAYAN

"Gemcitabine and cisplatin (GC) provide a similar survival advantage to methotrexate, vinblastine, doxorubicin and cisplatin (M-VAC) with a better safety profile and tolerability. This better-risk benefit ratio should change the standard of care for patients with locally advanced and metastatic transitional cell carcinoma from M-VAC to GC."[1]

Research Question: In patients with locally advanced or metastatic urothelial cell carcinoma (UCC), how does GC chemotherapy compare to M-VAC chemotherapy?

Funding: Eli Lilly and Company

Year Study Began: 1996

Year Study Published: 2000

Study Location: Canada, Denmark, Germany, Hungary, Italy, United Kingdom, Spain, Sweden

Who Was Studied: Patients with stage IV (histologically proven T4b, N2, N3, or M1) transitional UCC and no prior systemic chemotherapy

Who Was Excluded: Those with significant medical comorbidities such as active infection, any clinically significant cardiac arrhythmia, or class III congestive heart failure; also, pregnant women and those with central nervous system metastases or second primaries

Patients: 405

Study Overview:

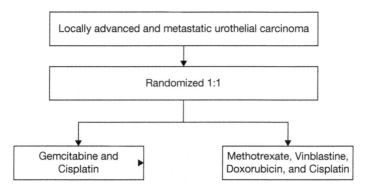

Study Intervention: GC (gemcitabine 1,000 mg/m^2 on days 1, 8, and 15; cisplatin 70 mg/m^2 on day 2) versus standard M-VAC every 28 days for a maximum of six cycles

Follow-up: Median length of follow-up: 19 months

Endpoints: Primary outcome: overall survival. Secondary outcomes: objective tumor response, duration of response, time to progressive disease, time to treatment failure, toxicity, change in performance status and weight, quality of life, and medical resource utilization.

RESULTS:

- Approximately 80% of patients were male; 70% of patients had documented metastatic disease and nearly half the patients had visceral metastases.
- Overall survival, time to progression, time to failure, and response rates were all similar (Table 28.1).
- Grade 4 anemia (3.5% vs. 2.1%) and thrombocytopenia (28.5% vs. 12.9%) were more common in the GC group, although transfusions were infrequent; grade 4 neutropenia (29.9% vs. 65.2%) and mucositis (4.2% vs. 0%) were more common in the M-VAC group.
- Drug-related mortality rates were 1% in the GC arm and 3% in the M-VAC arm.
- Medical resources per cycle of therapy related to hospitalization for febrile neutropenia strongly favored the GC group (9 admissions with 33 hospital days vs. 49 admissions with 272 hospital days).
- Quality of life appeared similar between the groups.

Table 28.1 ONCOLOGICAL OUTCOMES COMPARING SYSTEMIC GC TO M-VAC

	GC	M-VAC	Hazard Ratio (95% Confidence Interval)
Median overall survival (months)	13.8	14.8	1.04 (0.82 to 1.32)
Median time to progression (months)	7.4	7.4	1.05 (0.85 to 1.30)
Median time to failure (months)	5.8	4.6	0.89 (0.72 to 1.10)
Response rate (%)	49.4	45.7	0.97 (0.62 to 1.52)

Criticisms and Limitations: This was a superiority study with a negative result. While there were no statistically significant differences in oncological outcomes between groups, the confidence intervals were quite wide. Although the study has been interpreted as favoring GC over M-VAC in terms of a better toxicity profile, this was not reflected in the quality-of life-outcomes.

Other Relevant Studies and Information:

- An extension of this study with longer follow-up to 5 years found continued similar survival rates of 13.0% for GC and 15.3% for M-VAC (p = 0.53).[2]

- Current evidence-based guidelines of the European Association of Urology[3] recommend cisplatin-based chemotherapy in patients with metastatic UCC. GC and M-VAC are presented as being similarly effective.
- Carboplatin-based chemotherapy, on the other hand, results in inferior outcomes[4] and is reserved for patients unable to receive cisplatin.[3]

Summary and Implications: In patients with advanced bladder cancer, GC chemotherapy provides similar overall response rates, time to progression, and median survival when compared to M-VAC, with less grade 3 or 4 neutropenia, mucositis, and neutropenic fever/sepsis.

CLINICAL CASE: GC VERSUS M-VAC IN METASTATIC UROTHELIAL CARCINOMA

Case History:

A 50-year-old male is diagnosed with metastatic urothelial cell carcinoma of the bladder. A family friend died from bladder cancer 15 years ago and had been treated with chemotherapy, which he is very apprehensive about receiving given what he remembers from his friend's hospitalizations. How might this study aid in counseling this patient?

Suggested Answer:

This patient with advanced UCC should be offered platinum-based chemotherapy as a first-line option, assuming he has an appropriate functional status. Most centers now use GC regimens in lieu of M-VAC given its similar efficacy with an improved safety and adverse event profile, as this study demonstrated. The patient should still be carefully counseled on risks of therapy, including moderate to severe anemia and thrombocytopenia, nausea/vomiting, alopecia, need for hospitalization, and potential for treatment-related mortality.

References

1. von der Maase H, Hansen SW, Roberts JT, et al. Gemcitabine and cisplatin versus methotrexate, vinblastine, doxorubicin, and cisplatin in advanced or metastatic bladder cancer: results of a large, randomized, multinational, multicenter, phase III study. *J Clin Oncol* 2000;18(17):3068–77. doi: 10.1200/JCO.2000.18.17.3068 [published online first: 2000/09/23]

2. von der Maase H, Sengelov L, Roberts JT, et al. Long-term survival results of a randomized trial comparing gemcitabine plus cisplatin, with methotrexate, vinblastine, doxorubicin, plus cisplatin in patients with bladder cancer. *J Clin Oncol* 2005;23(21):4602–8. doi: 10.1200/JCO.2005.07.757 [published online first: 2005/07/22]

3. Witjes JA, Bruins HM, Cathomas R, et al. European Association of Urology guideline on muscle-invasive and metastatic bladder cancer 2020. Available from: https://uroweb.org/guideline/bladder-cancer-muscle-invasive-and-metastatic/#7. Accessed 2/25/2020.

4. Galsky MD, Chen GJ, Oh WK, et al. Comparative effectiveness of cisplatin-based and carboplatin-based chemotherapy for treatment of advanced urothelial carcinoma. *Ann Oncol* 2012;23(2):406–10. doi: 10.1093/annonc/mdr156 [published online first: 2011/05/06]

29

Pembrolizumab as Second-Line Therapy for Advanced Urothelial Carcinoma

KEYNOTE-045

PHILIPP DAHM AND VIKRAM M. NARAYAN

"Pembrolizumab was associated with significantly longer overall survival (by approximately 3 months) and with a lower rate of treatment-related adverse events than chemotherapy as second-line therapy for platinum-refractory advanced urothelial carcinoma."[1]

Research Question: In patients with advanced urothelial cancer that has recurred or progressed following platinum-based chemotherapy, how does pembrolizumab (an anti–PD-1 immunotherapy agent) compare to standard second-line agents (paclitaxel, docetaxel, or vinflunine)?

Funding: Merck

Year Study Began: 2014

Year Study Published: 2017

Study Location: 120 sites in 29 countries

Who Was Studied: Patients with histologically or cytologically confirmed urothelial carcinoma of the renal pelvis, ureter, bladder, or urethra that showed predominantly transitional-cell features with progression after platinum-based chemotherapy for advanced disease or recurrence within 12 months after the receipt of platinum-based adjuvant or neoadjuvant therapy for localized muscle-invasive disease. Patients also needed to have a performance-status score of 2 or less.

Who Was Excluded: Patients with a hemoglobin concentration of less than 10 g/dl, presence of liver metastases, and receipt of the last dose of most recent chemotherapy less than 3 months earlier. Also excluded were those who had received any prior anti–PD-1, anti–PD-L1, or anti–CTLA-4 therapy.

Patients: 542

Study Overview:

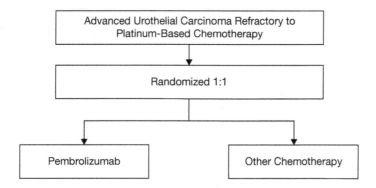

Study Interventions: Patients in the intervention arm received pembrolizumab (200 mg); patients in the control arm received investigator's choice of paclitaxel (175 mg/m^2), docetaxel (75 mg/m^2), or vinflunine (320 mg/m^2), all administered intravenously every 3 weeks.

Follow-up: The median duration of follow-up was 14.1 months (range 9.9 to 22.1 months).

Endpoints: Co-primary outcomes: overall survival and progression-free survival. Secondary endpoints: objective response rate (defined as complete or partial response) and duration of confirmed response as well adverse events.

RESULTS:

- The median patient age was approximately 66 years and the vast majority of patients had an Eastern Cooperative Oncology Group (ECOG) performance status of 0 or 1.
- 28.5% and 33.8% of the patients in the pembrolizumab arm and chemotherapy arm, respectively, had a tumor PD-L1 combined positive score of 10% or more.
- In the chemotherapy arm, approximately equally sized groups received docetaxel, paclitaxel, or vinflunine.
- Overall survival was significantly longer in the pembrolizumab group than in the chemotherapy group (hazard ratio [HR] 0.73; 95% confidence interval [CI], 0.59 to 0.91; p = 0.002); median overall survival was 10.3 months (95% CI, 8.0 to 11.8) in the pembrolizumab group, as compared with 7.4 months (95% CI, 6.1 to 8.3) in the chemotherapy group.
- There was no significant difference in the duration of progression-free survival between the pembrolizumab group and the chemotherapy group (HR 0.98; 95% CI, 0.81 to 1.19; p = 0.42).
- Overall survival and progression-free survival did not differ by PD-L1 status.
- Treatment-related events of grade 3, 4, or 5 severity were less frequent in the pembrolizumab group than in the chemotherapy group (15.0% vs. 49.4% of patients), as was treatment-related discontinuation of therapy (5.6% vs. 11.0%).

Criticism and Limitations: The study was stopped for benefit at the time of the second preplanned interim analysis, resulting in wider confidence intervals and potentially exaggerated effect sizes.[2] No platinum-containing second-line chemotherapy was compared against pembrolizumab; as a result, it is not clear how pembrolizumab compares to other second-line chemotherapy options.[3]

Other Relevant Studies and Information:

- Health-related quality-of-life outcomes were reported separately and appear to favor the pembrolizumab group.[4]
- Long-term results of KEYNOTE-045 were consistent with those of the primary analyses.[5]

- A cost-effectiveness analysis estimated the cost per quality-adjusted life year as $122,557.[6]
- On the basis of a single-armed trial (KEYNOTE-057), pembrolizumab was recently approved by the US Food and Drug Administration for high risk, non-muscle-invasive bladder cancer unresponsive to treatment with bacillus Calmette–Guérin (BCG).[7]

Summary and Implications: This study has ushered in the era of immune checkpoint inhibitors in the treatment of urothelial carcinoma. To date, pembrolizumab remains the only immune checkpoint inhibitor with a proven overall survival benefit over chemotherapy in a large randomized phase III trial. A number of additional agents such as nivolumab, durvalumab, and avelumab have since received regulatory approval, and a large number of trials are ongoing.[8]

CLINICAL CASE: PEMBROLIZUMAB AS SECOND-LINE TREATMENT FOR ADVANCED UROTHELIAL CARCINOMA

Case History:

A 72-year-old Caucasian man with a past medical history of tobacco dependence (>60 pack-year smoking history) and hypertension was diagnosed with T2HG urothelial carcinoma of the bladder approximately 6 months ago. Initial staging studies showed organ-confined disease with no evidence for hydronephrosis. Estimated glomerular filtration rate was more than 90 ml/min/1.73 m^2. He was counseled on treatment options and elected to undergo neoadjuvant chemotherapy (NAC) with dose-dense methotrexate, vinblastine, doxorubicin, and cisplatin (M-VAC) followed by planned radical cystectomy with urinary diversion. After two cycles of NAC, a restaging computed tomogram of the chest/abdomen/pelvis revealed new left external iliac lymphadenopathy and a 1.8-cm enlarged lymph node along the left common iliac artery. What is the next step?

Suggested Answer:

This scenario is concerning for disease progression while on platinum-based therapy. Current guidelines support the use of pembrolizumab in this setting (200 mg every 3 weeks for 24 months), regardless of the patient's PD-L1 expression status.[9] Patients should be carefully counseled on adverse events, and treating physicians should be particularly watchful for immune-related adverse events such as pneumonitis, colitis, and nephritis, which can be fatal if unrecognized and untreated. This patient could also be counseled on the risks and benefits of a lymph node biopsy to confirm disease progression, and evaluated for clinical trial enrollment, where available.

References

1. Bellmunt J, de Wit R, Vaughn DJ, et al. Pembrolizumab as second-line therapy for advanced urothelial carcinoma. *N Engl J Med* 2017;376(11):1015–26. doi: 10.1056/NEJMoa1613683 [published online first: 2017/02/18]
2. Bassler D, Briel M, Montori VM, et al. Stopping randomized trials early for benefit and estimation of treatment effects: systematic review and meta-regression analysis. *JAMA* 2010;303(12):1180–7. doi: 10.1001/jama.2010.310 [published online first: 2010/03/25]
3. Narayan V, Kahlmeyer A, Dahm P, et al. Pembrolizumab monotherapy versus chemotherapy for treatment of advanced urothelial carcinoma with disease progression during or following platinum-containing chemotherapy. A Cochrane Rapid Review. *Cochrane Database Syst Rev* 2018;7:CD012838. doi: 10.1002/14651858. CD012838.pub2 [published online first: 2018/07/24]
4. Vaughn DJ, Bellmunt J, Fradet Y, et al. Health-related quality-of-life analysis from KEYNOTE-045: a phase III study of pembrolizumab versus chemotherapy for previously treated advanced urothelial cancer. *J Clin Oncol* 2018;36(16):1579–87. doi: 10.1200/JCO.2017.76.9562 [published online first: 2018/03/29]
5. Fradet Y, Bellmunt J, Vaughn DJ, et al. Randomized phase III KEYNOTE-045 trial of pembrolizumab versus paclitaxel, docetaxel, or vinflunine in recurrent advanced urothelial cancer: results of >2 years of follow-up. *Ann Oncol* 2019;30(6):970–76. doi: 10.1093/annonc/mdz127 [published online first: 2019/05/06]
6. Sarfaty M, Hall PS, Chan KKW, et al. Cost-effectiveness of pembrolizumab in second-line advanced bladder cancer. *Eur Urol* 2018;74(1):57–62. doi: 10.1016/j.eururo.2018.03.006 [published online first: 2018/03/27]
7. US Food and Drug Administration. FDA approves pembrolizumab for BCG-unresponsive, high-risk non-muscle invasive bladder cancer. FDA approval notice, 2020. Available from: https://www.fda.gov/drugs/resources-information-approved-drugs/fda-approves-pembrolizumab-bcg-unresponsive-high-risk-non-muscle-invasive-bladder-cancer. Accessed 2/8/2020.
8. Gopalakrishnan D, Koshkin VS, Ornstein MC, et al. Immune checkpoint inhibitors in urothelial cancer: recent updates and future outlook. *Ther Clin Risk Manag* 2018;14:1019–40. doi: 10.2147/TCRM.S158753 [published online first: 2018/06/13]
9. Witjes JA, Bruins HM, Cathomas R, et al. European Association of Urology guideline on muscle-invasive and metastatic bladder cancer 2020. Available from: https://uroweb.org/guideline/bladder-cancer-muscle-invasive-and-metastatic/#7. Accessed 2/25/2020.

30

Cis-Diamminedichloroplatinum, Vinblastine, and Bleomycin Combination Chemotherapy in Disseminated Testicular Cancer

MICHAEL RISK

"We believe this regimen presents a major advance in the management of patients with disseminated testicular cancer."[1]

Research Question: What is the outcome of patients with disseminated testicular cancer treated with a three-drug combination consisting of cis-diamminedichloroplatinum, vinblastine, and bleomycin?

Funding: No information provided

Year Study Began: 1974

Year Study Published: September 1977

Study Location: Indiana University Medical Center

Who Was Studied: Consecutive patients with metastatic testicular germ cell tumor treated with a combination of bleomycin, vinblastine, and cisplatin

Who Was Excluded: Those who were refractory to one of the agents in the regimen given in a prior treatment, or those not treated with this combination. Three patients who died of disease within 2 weeks were excluded.

Patients: 47

Study Overview:

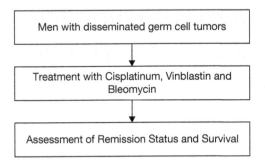

Study Interventions: Cisplatinum (20 mg/m^2) for 5 days every 3 weeks for three courses (total 9 weeks of therapy). Vinblastine (0.2 mg/kg) given on days 1 and 2 for a total of five courses every 3 weeks. Bleomycin (30 U) was given weekly for 12 weeks, with administration timed relative to vinblastine dose to promote synergism. Maintenance therapy was then given as a single 0.3-mg/kg injection of vinblastine every 4 weeks. Patients also received a scratch application of bacillus Calmette–Guérin (BCG) to the skin ("scarification") at the same interval for up to a total of 2 years.

Follow-up: Up to 30 months (median not reported)

Endpoints: Partial response was defined as a decrease of 50% or more in the sum of the diameters of all measurable lesions. Complete response was defined as complete resolution of all clinical, radiographic, and biochemical evidence of disease, including whole-lung tomograms and serum levels of beta subunit of human chorionic gonadotropin (hCG) and alpha fetoprotein (AFP).

RESULTS:

- Median patient age was 26 years (range 15 to 63); the disease stage ranged from elevated hCG levels only (n = 3) to advanced pulmonary disease (n = 9) and advanced abdominal disease (n = 9).

- All patients responded: 35 (74%) with clinical complete response and 12 (26%) with partial response. Of those with complete response to chemotherapy, 29 (83%) remained without evidence of disease at 6 to 30 months of follow-up.
- The likelihood of complete response correlated with burden of disease; it was 100% in those with marker elevation alone, 88% to 90% in the setting of minimal pulmonary disease with or without minimal abdominal disease, but only 55% to 67% in the setting of advanced pulmonary or abdominal disease.
- 5 of 12 partial responders achieved complete response with surgery.
- Major adverse effects of cisplatin included moderate to severe nausea and vomiting in all patients; nephrotoxicity, in particular prior to instituting aggressive intravenous hydration; and transient ototoxicity with high-frequency hearing loss.
- Major adverse effects of bleomycin included alopecia and weight loss; one patient died of pulmonary toxicity attributed to this agent.
- Major adverse effects of vinblastine included myalgia and bone marrow suppression; one patient with leukopenia was hospitalized for sepsis and ultimately died.

Criticism and Limitations: This was a single-arm study without a control group, so it is impossible to know how outcomes compared to alternative treatment approaches. The staging used is not as precise as the current models of clinical staging; thus, the stage or International Germ Cell Collaborative Group (IGCCCG) risk category of this patient population is unclear, making comparisons with other studies difficult. Computed tomography imaging was just emerging at the time of this study and was not part of routine staging.

Other Relevant Studies and Information:

- Prior studies found favorable response rates yet without long-term durability for the combination of vinblastine and bleomycin[2] as well as single-agent cisplatin.[3]
- An extension of this study with longer follow-up found that 25 of the 35 complete responders were alive and disease-free at greater than 10 years.[4]
- Later studies demonstrated that maintenance therapy had no effect on likelihood of relapse, and this practice has since been discontinued.[5]
- This trial also provided initial evidence on responsiveness based on disease stage; this is now stratified based on IGCCCG risk category.[6]

Summary and Implications: This study established that cisplatin-based combination chemotherapy was highly effective for patients with metastatic testicular cancer, representing a major advance in the treatment. Trials following this focused on improving cure rates as well as diminishing toxicity.

CLINICAL CASE: CISPLATINUM-BASED CHEMOTHERAPY IN ADVANCED TESTICULAR CANCER

Case History:

A 25-year-old man presents with low back pain and a left testicular mass, and ultrasound confirms a 6-cm heterogenous testicular mass. Serum tumor markers include AFP of 295 and hCG of 189. A computed tomogram of the chest, abdomen, and pelvis demonstrate two small pulmonary metastases as well as enlarged lymph nodes in the left retroperitoneum measuring about 3 cm. Orchiectomy demonstrates a non-seminoma. Serum markers are unchanged at 2 weeks after orchiectomy.

Suggested Answer:

This patient has a stage 3A testicular germ cell tumor, and since the publication of this trial cisplatin-based chemotherapy is the mainstay of treatment. As he has good-risk disease based on IGCCCG classification, current chemotherapy would typically be three cycles of bleomycin, etoposide, and cisplatin (BEP) or four cycles of etoposide and cisplatin (EP), followed by resection of residual masses larger than 1 cm if present. With this treatment in good-risk disease, 5-year overall survival exceeds 90%.

References

1. Einhorn LH, Donohue J. Cis-diamminedichloroplatinum, vinblastine, and bleomycin combination chemotherapy in disseminated testicular cancer. *Annals of Internal Medicine* 1977;87(3):293–8. [published online first: 1977/09/01]
2. Samuels ML, Holoye PY, Johnson DE. Bleomycin combination chemotherapy in the management of testicular neoplasia. *Cancer* 1975;36(2):318–26. [published online first: 1975/08/01]
3. Higby DJ, Wallace HJ, Jr., Albert D, et al. Diamminodichloroplatinum in the chemotherapy of testicular tumors. *Journal of Urology* 1974;112(1):100–4. [published online first: 1974/07/01]
4. Roth BJ, Greist A, Kubilis PS, et al. Cisplatin-based combination chemotherapy for disseminated germ cell tumors: long-term follow-up. *Journal of Clinical Oncology* 1988;6(8):1239–47. doi: 10.1200/jco.1988.6.8.1239 [published online first: 1988/08/01]

5. Einhorn LH, Williams SD, Troner M, et al. The role of maintenance therapy in disseminated testicular cancer. *New England Journal of Medicine* 1981;305(13):727–31. doi: 10.1056/nejm198109243051303 [published online first: 1981/09/24]

6. International Germ Cell Cancer Collaborative Group. International Germ Cell Consensus Classification: a prognostic factor-based staging system for metastatic germ cell cancers. *Journal of Clinical Oncology* 1997;15(2):594–603. doi: 10.1200/jco.1997.15.2.594 [published online first: 1997/02/01]

31

Treatment of Disseminated Germ Cell Tumors With Cisplatin, Bleomycin, and Either Vinblastine or Etoposide

PVB Versus BEP

MICHAEL RISK

"The BEP regimen substantially reduced neuromuscular toxicity and was therapeutically more effective in patients with advanced disease."[1]

Research Question: In patients with disseminated testicular cancer, how does treatment with cisplatin, etoposide, and bleomycin (BEP) compare to treatment with cisplatin, vinblastine, and bleomycin (PVB)?

Funding: National Institute of Health and Cancer Center grants

Year Study Began: 1982

Year Study Published: June 1987

Study Location: Multicenter cooperative group trial performed at 24 institutions

Who Was Studied: Patients with metastatic germ cell tumors from any primary site, including testicular or extragonadal. Patients with seminoma were eligible only if radiation treatment was considered inappropriate.

Who Was Excluded: Patients previously treated with any study drug

Patients: 244 (121 with PVB, 123 with BEP)

Study Overview:

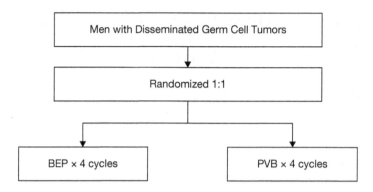

Study Interventions: Cisplatinum (20 mg/m^2) daily for 5 days every 3 weeks for four courses. Bleomycin (30 U) was given on days 2, 9, and 16 of each cycle. For those in the PVB arm, vinblastine (0.15 mg/kg) given on days 1 and 2, while those in the BEP arm received etoposide (100 mg/m^2) on days 1 to 5. In patients with prior radiotherapy and those developing granulocytopenia and fever, doses were reduced. Bleomycin was discontinued if there was any evidence of pulmonary fibrosis.

Follow-up: Median follow-up was 90 weeks.

Endpoints: Complete clinical response was determined by resolution of all visible disease on computed tomography and normalization of tumor markers. Those who underwent surgery for residual disease and were found to have only necrosis/fibrosis were also considered to have had a complete response.

Patients found to have mature teratoma at the time of surgery were considered partial remissions, and those with immature teratoma were categorized as disease-free (with teratoma).

RESULTS:

- The most common histology types were teratocarcinoma (36.5%), embryonal carcinoma (36.1%), and seminoma (16.8%); the distribution

by disease extent of minimal, moderate, and advanced was 46.7%, 23.8%, and 29.5%, respectively.
- 74 patients in each arm (61% PVB, 60% BEP) had a complete response to induction chemotherapy.
- Chemotherapy and surgery led to clinical disease-free status for 74% in the PVB group versus 83% in the BEP group.
- 15 recurrences happened overall, with no significant difference between the regimens (9 PVB vs. 6 BEP).
  - 12 occurred in those with a complete response.
  - 11 of the 15 occurred within the first year from treatment.
- Overall survival was about 80% at 2 years in both regimens.
- Subset analysis of those classified as having advanced disease showed significantly improved survival with BEP compared to PVB.
- Neuromuscular toxicity was less with BEP compared to PVB.
  - Paresthesias: 38% PVB versus 23% BEP
  - Abdominal cramps: 20% PVB versus 5% BEP
  - Myalgias: 19% PVB versus 1% BEP
- Other adverse events were similar between the two regimens, with 12 drug-related deaths overall (7 in the PVB arm, 5 in the BEP arm).

Criticism and Limitations: This was a relatively small study that enrolled patients of different risk categories by today's standards. It also predates modern staging techniques using computed tomography, which limits generalizability.

Other Relevant Studies and Information:

- Prior studies had suggested a role for etoposide as salvage therapy in germ cell tumors previously treated with other chemotherapy regimens.[2]
- Subsequent studies have since demonstrated that those with favorable disease characteristics (all metastatic seminoma and select non-seminomas with modest marker elevations and absence of non-pulmonary, visceral metastases), currently termed "good risk" according to International Germ Cell Collaborative Group (IGCCCG) classification,[3] can be treated with three cycles of BEP instead of four with no decrease in efficacy.[4]
- Based on current guidelines, BEP has become the "workhorse" of systemic chemotherapy for patients with advanced testicular cancer; guidelines include tailoring the number of cycles to the disease extent.[5,6]

Summary and Implications: This study demonstrated BEP to be superior to PVB in terms of adverse effects, with at least equivalent efficacy if not superiority in the setting of advanced disease. This study established what continues to be the standard induction chemotherapy regimen used for the majority of patients with metastatic testicular cancer.[5,6]

CLINICAL CASE: BEP CHEMOTHERAPY IN POOR-RISK NON-SEMINOMA

Case History:

A 25-year-old male presents with shortness of breath worsening over the past month, and physical exam demonstrates a large right testicular mass. Computed tomographic evaluation demonstrates large-volume pulmonary and retroperitoneal masses. He undergoes retroperitoneal mass biopsy, which demonstrates metastatic germ cell tumor. Serum markers are notable for significant elevation of human chorionic gonadotropin (hCG) to 110,000.

Suggested Answer:

This patient has poor-risk non-seminoma, demonstrated by the elevated hCG above 50,000.[3] Given his symptomatic pulmonary metastasis, retroperitoneal biopsy to confirm germ cell tumor is reasonable, along with proceeding directly to induction chemotherapy with orchiectomy deferred until completion of treatment. The chemotherapy options in this setting include four cycles of BEP or four cycles of VIP (etoposide, ifosfamide, and cisplatin), with the majority of patients undergoing four cycles of BEP, which was established in this trial as efficacious in advanced disease.[5,6] Four cycles of VIP does not provide an increased likelihood of cure as first-line therapy but is mainly used if there is concern for bleomycin toxicity,[7] which may be a consideration given his respiratory symptoms.

References

1. Williams SD, Birch R, Einhorn LH, et al. Treatment of disseminated germ-cell tumors with cisplatin, bleomycin, and either vinblastine or etoposide. *N Engl J Med* 1987;316(23):1435–40. doi: 10.1056/nejm198706043162302 [published online first: 1987/06/04]
2. Williams SD, Einhorn LH, Greco FA, et al. VP-16-213 salvage therapy for refractory germinal neoplasms. *Cancer* 1980;46(10):2154–8. [published online first: 1980/11/15]

3. International Germ Cell Cancer Collaborative Group. International Germ Cell Consensus Classification: a prognostic factor-based staging system for metastatic germ cell cancers. *J Clin Oncol* 1997;15(2):594–603. doi: 10.1200/jco.1997.15.2.594 [published online first: 1997/02/01]

4. Saxman SB, Finch D, Gonin R, et al. Long-term follow-up of a phase III study of three versus four cycles of bleomycin, etoposide, and cisplatin in favorable-prognosis germ-cell tumors: the Indiana University experience. *J Clin Oncol* 1998;16(2):702–6. doi: 10.1200/jco.1998.16.2.702 [published online first: 1998/02/20]

5. Albers P, Albrecht W, Algaba F, et al. Guidelines on testicular cancer: 2015 update. *Eur Urol* 2015;68(6):1054–68. doi: 10.1016/j.eururo.2015.07.044 [published online first: 2015/08/25]

6. Stephenson A, Eggener SE, Bass EB, et al. Diagnosis and treatment of early stage testicular cancer: AUA guideline. *J Urol* 2019;202(2):272–81. doi: 10.1097/JU.0000000000000318 [published online first: 2019/05/07]

7. Hinton S, Catalano PJ, Einhorn LH, et al. Cisplatin, etoposide and either bleomycin or ifosfamide in the treatment of disseminated germ cell tumors: final analysis of an intergroup trial. *Cancer* 2003;97(8):1869–75. doi: 10.1002/cncr.11271 [published online first: 2003/04/04]

32

Urinary Volume, Water Intake, and Stone Recurrence in Idiopathic Calcium Nephrolithiasis

A 5-Year Randomized Prospective Study

MICHAEL S. BOROFSKY AND VINCENT G. BIRD

"We conclude that urine volume is a real stone risk factor in nephrolithiasis and that a large intake of water is the initial therapy for the prevention of stone recurrences."[1]

Research Question: In patients with idiopathic calcium nephrolithiasis, does increased water intake prevent stone recurrences?

Funding: No information provided

Year Study Began: 1986

Year Study Published: 1996

Study Location: University of Parma, Italy

Who Was Studied: Patients with one prior episode of idiopathic calcium nephrolithiasis (with chemical analysis showing calcium oxalate stone with or without traces of calcium phosphate) that had resolved by spontaneous stone passage or had been treated with shockwave lithotripsy, percutaneous techniques, or other procedures

Who Was Excluded: Patients with residual stone disease (as determined by ultrasound or intravenous pyelogram), hypertension, or other diseases that required particular dietary measures or drug therapy

Patients: 220

Study Overview:

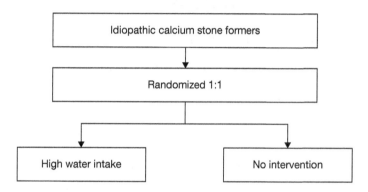

Study Interventions: Patients in the intervention arm were instructed to titrate their water intake to a daily urine output of at least 2 liters and asked to measure their urine volume every 2 to 3 months. Patients in the control arm were not given any specific instructions. In both groups a 24-hour urine collection was performed. Patients were asked to report any episodes of renal colic or stone passage. On an annual basis ultrasound and/or plain x-rays were performed.

Follow-up: 5 years

Endpoints: Stone recurrence at 5 years, time to stone recurrence, 24-hour urine parameters (there was no prespecified primary outcome)

RESULTS:

- Enrolled patients were approximately 41 years old and approximately two-thirds were men.
- During the 5-year follow-up period, 12 of the 99 patients in the intervention arm and 27 of the 100 patients in the control arm presented

with recurrent stones; risk ratio 0.45 (95% confidence interval, 0.24 to 0.83).

- Time to stone recurrence was longer in the intervention arm ($p = 0.006$); in those patients who passed a stone, time to recurrence was 38.7 ± 13.2 months in the intervention arm and 25.1 ± 16.4 months in the control arm ($p = 0.016$).
- Urinary stone risk measured as calcium oxalate and calcium phosphate supersaturation was lower in the intervention group.

Criticism and Limitations:

- This study focuses on the role of secondary stone prevention for calcium oxalate and phosphate stone formers with a single prior stone episode; it does not address primary prevention or the impact of increased fluid intake in individuals who have had multiple stones or other types of stones.
- The study predates modern imaging technology for stone disease using computed tomography and relied entirely on ultrasound and plain x-rays in identifying recurrent stone formers.
- It is unclear from the reported study what percentage of patients presented with symptoms of renal colic versus asymptomatic stone disease and in what location of the kidney.
- The study also does not provide information about participants' consumption of other non-water beverages; this matters, as certain types of beverages, such as coffee, teas, juices, and soda, are known to have potentially different effects on urinary stone risk.[2]
- Actual fluid consumption was not measured, yet reported urine volumes in the intervention groups were high at 2.7 liters in the fifth year of follow-up. This degree of compliance is unusually high and stands in contrast with other studies indicating that long-term patient compliance with medical and dietary recommendations to prevent kidney stones is often suboptimal.[3,4]

Other Relevant Studies and Information:

- The Health Professionals Follow-Up Study[5] and the Nurses' Health Study I[6] were large observational studies that both supported an important role for increased fluid intake to reduce the risk of stone recurrence.

- Fluid intake could have a major economic impact on reducing the societal costs of nephrolithiasis. Models based on the French healthcare system estimate that increased fluid therapy could prevent over 11,000 stone events per year, leading to a savings of nearly 50 million euros.[7]
- A systematic review found increased fluid intake to be the only intervention of proven benefit in individuals with one prior episode of calcium nephrolithiasis.[8]

Summary and Implications: High water intake to generate urine output of over 2 liters per day is associated with a decreased risk of stone recurrence in first-time calcium oxalate stone formers. It also reduces the urinary supersaturation of multiple crystal types responsible for stone formation.

CLINICAL CASE: INCREASED WATER INTAKE FOR SECONDARY STONE PREVENTION

Case History:
A 35-year-old man is seen for outpatient follow-up after a first episode of renal colic with spontaneous passage of a 4-mm ureteral stone. Stone analysis reveals 90% calcium oxalate and 10% calcium phosphate. What recommendation can be given to reduce his risk of recurrent stones?

Suggested Answer:
This trial demonstrated a decreased risk of stone recurrence among first-time calcium oxalate stone formers who were advised and adhered to a high-fluid diet and were able to achieve greater than 2 liters of urine output per day. The patient should be advised to measure his urine at home to ensure he is taking in sufficient amounts of water to produce at least 2 liters of urine per day, as this may vary depending on environmental and occupational exposures and insensate water losses. Because patients in this study achieved an even greater mean urine output than 2 liters (2.1 to 2.6, depending on the year), 2.5 liters of urine output per day may be optimal to decrease the risk of recurrence, as reflected by guidelines from the American Urological Association, the European Association of Urology, and the American College of Physicians.[6,9,10]

References

1. Borghi L, Meschi T, Schianchi T, et al. Urine volume: stone risk factor and preventive measure. *Nephron* 1999;81(Suppl 1):31–7. doi: 10.1159/000046296 [published online first: 1999/01/05 21:58]

2. Ticinesi A, Nouvenne A, Borghi L, et al. Water and other fluids in nephrolithiasis: state of the art and future challenges. *Crit Rev Food Sci Nutr* 2017;57(5):963–74. doi: 10.1080/10408398.2014.964355 [published online first: 2015/05/16]

3. Khambati A, Matulewicz RS, Perry KT, et al. Factors associated with compliance to increased fluid intake and urine volume following dietary counseling in first-time kidney stone patients. *J Endourol* 2017;31(6):605–10. doi: 10.1089/end.2016.0836 [published online first: 2017/03/21]

4. Ortiz-Alvarado O, Miyaoka R, Kriedberg C, et al. Impact of dietary counseling on urinary stone risk parameters in recurrent stone formers. *J Endourol* 2011;25(3):535–40. doi: 10.1089/end.2010.0241 [published online first: 2011/03/03]

5. Curhan GC, Willett WC, Rimm EB, et al. A prospective study of dietary calcium and other nutrients and the risk of symptomatic kidney stones. *N Engl J Med* 1993;328(12):833–8. doi: 10.1056/NEJM199303253281203 [published online first: 1993/03/25]

6. Pearle MS, Goldfarb DS, Assimos DG, et al. Medical management of kidney stones: AUA guideline. *J Urol* 2014;192(2):316–24. doi: 10.1016/j.juro.2014.05.006 [published online first: 2014/05/27]

7. Lotan Y, Pearle MS. Cost-effectiveness of primary prevention strategies for nephrolithiasis. *J Urol* 2011;186(2):550–5. doi: 10.1016/j.juro.2011.03.133 [published online first: 2011/06/21]

8. Fink HA, Wilt TJ, Eidman KE, et al. Medical management to prevent recurrent nephrolithiasis in adults: a systematic review for an American College of Physicians clinical guideline. *Ann Intern Med* 2013;158(7):535–43. doi: 10.7326/0003-4819-158-7-201304020-00005 [published online first: 2013/04/03]

9. Skolarikos A, Straub M, Knoll T, et al. Metabolic evaluation and recurrence prevention for urinary stone patients: EAU guidelines. *Eur Urol* 2015;67(4):750–63. doi: 10.1016/j.eururo.2014.10.029 [published online first: 2014/12/03]

10. Qaseem A, Fink HA, Denberg TD. Prevention of recurrent nephrolithiasis in adults. *Ann Intern Med* 2015;162(7):529. doi: 10.7326/L15-5074-3 [published online first: 2015/04/07]

33

A Prospective Study of Dietary Calcium and Other Nutrients and the Risk of Symptomatic Kidney Stones

MICHAEL S. BOROFSKY AND VINCENT G. BIRD

"These prospective data provide no support for the belief that higher consumption of calcium from dietary sources increases the risk of symptomatic kidney stones; in fact, the data suggest that the relation may actually be inverse."[1]

Research Question: In individuals without a history of nephrolithiasis, how is dietary calcium intake associated with the risk of symptomatic stone disease?

Funding: National Institutes of Health and American Kidney Fund

Year Study Began: 1986

Year Study Published: 1993

Study Location: United States

Who Was Studied: Male healthcare professionals aged 40 to 75 years without prior history of stone disease enrolled in the Health Professionals Follow-up Study[2]

Who Was Excluded: Men with a history of nephrolithiasis

Patients: 45,619

Study Overview:

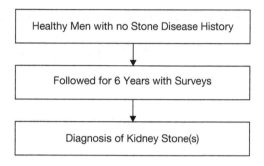

Study Interventions: This was a prospective cohort study without a specific intervention or comparison group. At the beginning of the study in 1986, participating men were asked to complete a validated semi-quantitative food-frequency questionnaire about the average use of 131 foods and beverages during the previous year. Participants also provided information on their state of residence, weight, height, and use of thiazide diuretics. Their level of physical activity was calculated based on the reported frequency and duration of various forms of exercise. Two and 6 years later, they were mailed follow-up questionnaires asking to report any new diagnosis of kidney stones since the initiation of the study. Dietary calcium intake was analyzed using quintiles.

Follow-up: 6 years

Endpoints: Primary outcome: new kidney stone diagnosis accompanied by pain or hematuria. Secondary outcomes: none.

RESULTS:

- During over 165,090 person-years, 505 cases of new stones occurred.
- Mean daily dietary calcium was lower in the group who formed stones compared to those who did not (797 ± 280 mg vs. 851 ± 307 mg) (p < 0.01).
- High daily dietary calcium intake was strongly associated with decreased risk of stones after adjusting for covariates (p < 0.01).

- Relative risk of stone in the group with the highest calcium intake compared to the lowest was 0.56 (95% confidence interval [CI], 0.43 to 0.73).
- There was no difference in urinary sodium levels or percentages of men taking calcium supplements or thiazide diuretics between groups.
- No significant association was found between use of calcium supplements and risk of kidney stone.

Criticism and Limitations: Findings in this study were obtained from a cohort of male patients over the age of 40 and may not be directly applicable to younger or female patients. Dietary calcium intake was estimated based on a validated dietary questionnaire; however, as the authors themselves admit, this may not correspond perfectly with actual dietary intake. Only 71.5% had calcium-containing stones, and there was no discrimination between calcium oxalate and calcium phosphate stones, for which dietary calcium intake may play a different role. The inclusion of non-calcium stone types may have potentially decreased the inverse association observed with dietary calcium intake. Lastly, the high rate of uric acid stones (23%) stands out in comparison to other large cross-sectional studies that had a reported prevalence of 7% to 14%.[3]

Other Relevant Studies and Information:

- A subsequent study replicated these study findings of the association between increased dietary calcium and decreased risk of kidney stones in the all-female Nurses' Health Studies I and II.[4,5]
- A subsequent randomized control trial confirmed that low dietary calcium intake is associated with an increased risk of kidney stones.[6] Patients adhering to a normal-calcium diet (1,200 mg/day) had a lower relative risk of 0.49 (05% CI, 0.24 to 0.98, p = 0.04) for kidney stone formation compared to patients on a low-calcium diet (400 mg/day).
- Recommendations for moderate dietary calcium intake (1,000 to 1,200 mg/day) rather than reducing intake has since become a guideline recommendation for metabolic stone management by both the American Urological Association[7] and the European Association of Urology.[8]

Summary and Implications: This study found that increased dietary calcium intake did not promote clinical stone disease.

CLINICAL CASE: DIETARY COUNSELING FOR PREVENTION OF CALCIUM STONES

Case History:

A 50-year-old, first-time calcium oxalate stone former seeks dietary counseling to reduce the likelihood of stone recurrence. Based on the results of this study, how would you counsel this patient?

Suggested Answer:

The results of the study demonstrated a 0.56 relative risk of stone formation in the cohort of men who took in the highest as opposed to lowest amounts of dietary calcium. As such, the patient should be counseled that he should not avoid dietary calcium and rather should maintain moderate dietary calcium intake (between 1,000 and 1,200 mg/day).

References

1. Curhan GC, Willett WC, Rimm EB, Stampfer MJ. A prospective study of dietary calcium and other nutrients and the risk of symptomatic kidney stones. *N Engl J Med.* 1993;328(12):833–8.

2. Rimm EB, Giovannucci EL, Willett WC, et al. Prospective study of alcohol consumption and risk of coronary disease in men. *Lancet.* 1991;338(8765):464–8.

3. Xu G, Wen J, Wang B, et al. The clinical efficacy and safety of ureteroscopic laser papillotomy to treat intraductal papillary calculi associated with medullary sponge kidney. *Urology.* 2015;86(3):472–6.

4. Curhan GC, Willett WC, Speizer FE, et al. Comparison of dietary calcium with supplemental calcium and other nutrients as factors affecting the risk for kidney stones in women. *Ann Intern Med.* 1997;126(7):497–504.

5. Curhan GC, Willett WC, Knight EL, Stampfer MJ. Dietary factors and the risk of incident kidney stones in younger women: Nurses' Health Study II. *Arch Intern Med.* 2004;164(8):885–91.

6. Borghi L, Schianchi T, Meschi T, et al. Comparison of two diets for the prevention of recurrent stones in idiopathic hypercalciuria. *N Engl J Med.* 2002;346(2):77–84.

7. Pearle MS, Goldfarb DS, Assimos DG, et al. Medical management of kidney stones: AUA guideline. *J Urol.* 2014;192(2):316–24.

8. Skolarikos A, Straub M, Knoll T, et al. Metabolic evaluation and recurrence prevention for urinary stone patients: EAU guidelines. *Eur Urol.* 2015;67(4):750–63.

9. Prochaska ML, Taylor EN, Curhan GC. Insights into nephrolithiasis from the Nurses' Health Studies. *Am J Public Health.* 2016;106(9):1638–43.

First Clinical Experience With Extracorporeally Induced Destruction of Kidney Stones by Shock Waves

MICHAEL S. BOROFSKY AND VINCENT G. BIRD

"It can be concluded that noninvasive treatment of patients with kidney stones by high-energy shock waves is efficient. However, shock wave treatment of renal calculi is in its early stage of evolution. Therefore, the ultimate potential of this method cannot be defined precisely in its present development."[1]

Research Question: In patients with kidney stones, does extracorporeal shock wave lithotripsy result in stone fragmentation and stone passage?

Funding: Supported in part by a grant by the German Ministry of Research and Technology

Year Study Began: Not reported

Year Study Published: 1982

Study Location: University of Munich, Germany

Who Was Studied: Patients with renal stones

Who Was Excluded: Patients with intrarenal obstruction. Initially also patients with cardiopulmonary problem and those with urinary tract infections.

Patients: 72

Study Overview:

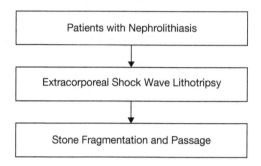

Study Interventions: This was a case series of patients with renal stones treated with extracorporeal shock wave lithotripsy (ESWL) within 12 months; there was no comparison group. Patients were treated with an early spark electrode lithotripter model in a water bath. The procedure took 30 to 45 minutes, was performed mostly under peridural anesthesia, and included the application of 500 to 1,000 shocks of 0.5-microsecond duration.

Follow-up: Not reported

Endpoints: Stone fragmentation, stone passage, renal clearance before and after ESWL and additional stone treatment (there was no prespecified primary outcome)

RESULTS:

- 40% of patients had a prior history of open stone surgery.
- Clinical follow-up was available for 63 patients, of whom 59 had a stone in the renal pelvis or calyx; 2 had staghorn calculi and 2 had ureteral stones.
- Among the 59 patients with stones in the renal pelvis or calyx, 91.5% (54/59) had fragments of 1 to 2 mm in size and 8.5% (5/59) had larger residual stones, often in the lower pole, but of a size amenable to spontaneous passage.

- A total of six patients underwent secondary surgical intervention; this included the two patients with staghorn calculi and two patients with ureteral stones.
- 15% of patients suffered symptoms of renal colic.
- Average renal clearance of the treated kidney was similar before and after ESWL.

Criticism and Limitations: This study represents an uncontrolled case series of patients with renal stones treated with ESWL without a comparison group. It lacks well-defined inclusion/exclusion criteria with regard to stone type, location, or size, and short-term follow-up is only available for a subset of patients.

Other Relevant Studies and Information:

- A number of randomized controlled trials have compared ESWL to the two competing treatment modalities for renal stones, namely percutaneous nephrolithotomy and ureteroscopy.[2,3] ESWL has the least morbidity but is also the treatment modality most likely to require retreatment. It does not appear to cause any long-term adverse effects.[4]
- The Lower Pole study I has informed the comparative effectiveness of ESWL versus percutaneous nephrolithotomy for lower-pole nephrolithiasis, with ESWL having lower morbidity but also lower stone-free rates.[5]
- Skin-to-stone distance, bone density, and stone density as assessed by Hounsfield units are the most important predictors of outcome aside from stone size and location.[6]

Summary and Implications: This case series provides the first structured report of the initial clinical experience with ESWL for renal (and ureteral) stone disease. ESWL continues to be an important treatment option for both renal and ureteral stones up to 20 mm in size based on current evidence-based guidelines.[7,8]

CLINICAL CASE: ESWL FOR RENAL STONES

Case History:
A 56-year-old male is incidentally found to have a 14-mm stone in the left renal pelvis. He denies any history of urinary tract infection and his urinalysis is unremarkable. He has normal renal function and no history of a bleeding disorder.

Stone density based on a computed tomography scan is 570 Hounsfield units, the patient has a normal body habitus, and his skin-to-stone distance is 7 cm. How should he be treated?

Suggested Answer:

Because the patient's stone is larger than 10 mm, it is unlikely to pass spontaneously and is likely to grow further and become the potential source of complications such as pain, obstruction, infection, and ultimately loss of renal function; therefore, treatment is recommended.[8] American Urology Association guidelines recommend ESWL as the procedure with the least degree of morbidity and lowest rate of complications, but it may have to be repeated in order for the patient to become stone-free. The alternative would be primary ureteroscopy and laser lithotripsy, which has a higher success rates but is also more invasive and may leave the patient with a temporary ureteral stent. That being said, based on stone density, location, and body habitus, this patient appears a very good ESWL candidate and may achieve stone freedom in single setting.

References

1. Chaussy C, Schmiedt E, Jocham D, et al. First clinical experience with extracorporeally induced destruction of kidney stones by shock waves. *J Urol.* 1982;127(3):417–20.
2. Matlaga BR, Jansen JP, Meckley LM, et al. Treatment of ureteral and renal stones: a systematic review and meta-analysis of randomized, controlled trials. *J Urol.* 2012;188(1):130–7.
3. Srisubat A, Potisat S, Lojanapiwat B, et al. Extracorporeal shock wave lithotripsy (ESWL) versus percutaneous nephrolithotomy (PCNL) or retrograde intrarenal surgery (RIRS) for kidney stones. *Cochrane Database Syst Rev.* 2014(11):CD007044.
4. Turk C, Petrik A, Sarica K, et al. EAU guidelines on interventional treatment for urolithiasis. *Eur Urol.* 2016;69(3):475–82.
5. Albala DM, Assimos DG, Clayman RV, et al. Lower pole I: a prospective randomized trial of extracorporeal shock wave lithotripsy and percutaneous nephrostolithotomy for lower pole nephrolithiasis—initial results. *J Urol.* 2001;166(6):2072–80.
6. Pareek G, Hedican SP, Lee FT, Jr., Nakada SY. Shock wave lithotripsy success determined by skin-to-stone distance on computed tomography. *Urology.* 2005;66(5):941–4.
7. National Institute for Health and Care Excellence. Renal and ureteric stones: assessment and management. *BJU Int.* 2019;123(2):220–32.
8. Assimos D, Krambeck A, Miller NL, et al. Surgical management of stones: American Urological Association/Endourological Society guideline, part I. *J Urol.* 2016;196(4):1153–60.

Shock Wave Lithotripsy Versus Ureteroscopy for Lower-Pole Caliceal Calculi 1 cm or Less

VINCENT G. BIRD AND MICHAEL S. BOROFSKY

"This study failed to demonstrate a statistically significant difference in stone-free rates between SWL and URS for the treatment of small lower pole renal calculi."[1]

Research Question: In patients with lower-pole stones 1 cm and less, how does shock wave lithotripsy (SWL) compare to retrograde ureteroscopy (URS)?

Funding: Supported by Boston Scientific, Natick, Massachusetts

Year Study Began: 2000

Year Study Published: 2005

Study Location: 19 medical centers in the United States and Canada

Who Was Studied: Adult patients with isolated lower-pole stones 1 cm or less in size in whom treatment was indicated (due to pain, infection, hematuria, local obstruction, and/or stone growth)

Who Was Excluded: Patients with concomitant same-side, non–lower-pole stones; ureteral strictures; ureteropelvic junction obstruction; infundibular stenosis; renal disease (serum creatinine more than 3 mg/dl); pregnancy; previous failed treatment; or an active infection

Patients: 78

Study Overview:
Prospective, randomized, multicenter trial in adult patients

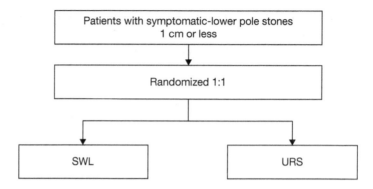

Study Interventions: SWL versus ureteroscopy and stone retrieval or intracorporeal lithotripsy. The choice of SWL device was based on the availability at the enrolling institution; nine different types of lithotriptors were used in the study. The power settings and number of shocks administered were left to the discretion of the treating physician. A variety of ureteroscopes was used based on the availability at the local institution. Dilation of the intramural ureter was performed as needed; the use of access sheaths, method of stone retrieval, and stent placement (or not) were left to the investigators' discretion.

Follow-Up: Initial follow-up occurred 2 to 6 weeks after treatment to document any retreatments and 3 months for stone-free rate (SFR).

Endpoints: Primary endpoint: SFR at 3 months by computed tomographic imaging. Secondary endpoints: quality-of-life data using the RAND 36-Item Health Survey, pain assessment, and time to return to work/normal activity.

RESULTS:

- Of 78 randomized patients, 11 were excluded, leaving 67 patients (32 for SWL and 35 for URS) in the outcome analyses.

- A ureteral stent was placed in 89% of patients (31/35) after URS. Only one patient undergoing SWL received a stent at the time of treatment. Three SWL patients had preexisting stents.
- All patients treated with SWL and 94% treated with URS were discharged home the day of treatment.
- Radiographic follow-up for the primary endpoint of SFR was available for only 52 of 78 randomized patients (66.7%). Nine of the 26 patients (35%) in the SWL arm and 16 of the 32 patients (50%) in the URS arm were stone-free. The risk ratio was 0.69 (95% confidence interval [CI], 0.37 to 1.30).
- Secondary treatments were necessary in 5 SWL cases and 2 URS cases; risk ratio of 2.7 (95% CI, 0.57 to 12.68).
- Six patients per group returned to the emergency room visit postoperatively. None of the patients treated with SWL but 3 patients with URS required hospitalization.
- Patients with SWL required significantly fewer pain pills postoperatively than those treated with URS.
- Complications for both groups were reported as infrequent and of low severity.
- 90% of patients who underwent SWL versus 63% of those who underwent URS indicated that they would choose to undergo the same procedure again (p = 0.031).

Criticisms and Limitations: The study has a number of limitations, such as lack of blinding and a large proportion of patients randomized but not included in the final analyses. Since that time, URS technology has evolved considerably; ureteroscopes with smaller caliber, better optical qualities, and better deflection abilities[2] have become available, thereby limiting the generalizability of the findings. The authors concluded that there was no statistically significant difference in the stone-free rates; however, that conclusion is tempered by the low event rates and resulting wide confidence intervals.

Other Relevant Studies and Information:
- A large number of urologists now consider URS first-line treatment for the types of stones described in this study.[3]
- Based on the findings of this study, both American Urological Association and European Association of Urology guidelines endorse renal stone treatment with URS or SWL,[4,5] but they also clearly point

out that URS has undergone significant evolution and is now often preferred.

Summary and Implications: This study suggested that there is little to no difference in stone-free rates with SWL versus URS for the treatment of small lower-pole renal calculi. As it requires few repeat procedures for treating residual stones, URS is now widely embraced by urologists for this indication. However, a potential tradeoff is a higher degree of invasiveness compared to SWL.

CLINICAL CASE: SWL VERSUS URS FOR SMALL LOWER-POLE CALICEAL STONE

Case History:

A 36-year-old female is found to have recurrent stone disease noted on recent imaging. Her previous stones have been calcium oxalate monohydrate. She states that she travels internationally for business regularly and does not want to risk experiencing ureteral colic on one of her upcoming trips abroad. Physical exam reveals an obese female with a body mass index (BMI) of 36. Findings on urine and serum analysis are all within normal limits; there is no evidence of infection. Computed tomography shows a 9-mm right lower-pole stone measuring 1,410 Hounsfield units; the stone-to-skin distance is 14 cm. She asks about the most efficacious treatment option.

Suggested Answer:

Based on the current best evidence that is provided by this randomized controlled trial, both SWL and URS would appear to be options for treating her right lower-pole stone. However, both the high density of the stone and the stone-to-skin distance of 14 cm are relative contraindications for SWL. Targeting the stone radiographically may be difficult and fragmentation might be inadequate, requiring retreatment. Especially in a patient like her seeking expeditious treatment, URS with laser storm fragmentation and basketing of fragments is the preferred option.

References

1. Pearle MS, Lingeman JE, Leveillee R, et al. Prospective, randomized trial comparing shock wave lithotripsy and ureteroscopy for lower pole caliceal calculi 1 cm or less. *J Urol.* 2005;173(6):2005–9.

2. Chew BH, Lange D. The future of ureteroscopy. *Minerva Urol Nefrol.* 2016 Dec;68(6):592–7.

3. Dauw CA, Simeon L, Alruwaily AF, et al. Contemporary practice patterns of flexible ureteroscopy for treating renal stones: results of a worldwide survey. *J Endourol.* 2015 Nov;29(11):1221–30.

4. Assimos D, Krambeck A, Miller NL, et al. Surgical management of stones: American Urological Association/Endourological Society guideline, part I. *J Urol.* 2016 Oct;196(4):1153–60.

5. Türk C, Petřík A, Sarica K, et al. EAU guidelines on interventional treatment for urolithiasis. *Eur Urol.* 2016 Mar;69(3):475–82.

36

Extracorporeal Shock Wave Lithotripsy Versus Percutaneous Nephrolithotomy for Lower-Pole Nephrolithiasis

The Lower Pole I Study

VINCENT G. BIRD AND MICHAEL S. BOROFSKY

"Stone clearance from the lower pole following shock wave lithotripsy is poor, especially for stones greater than 10 mm. in diameter. Calculi greater than 10 mm. in diameter are better managed initially with percutaneous removal due to its high degree of efficacy and acceptably low morbidity."[1]

Research Question: How does extracorporeal shock wave lithotripsy (ESWL) compare to percutaneous nephrolithotomy (PCNL) for the treatment of symptomatic lower-pole renal calculi?

Funding: Microvasive

Year Study Began: 1998

Year Study Published: 2001

Study Location: Numerous sites in the United States, with an additional site each in Canada and Mexico

Who Was Studied: Patients older than 18 years with symptomatic lower-pole calculi 3.0 cm or less in aggregate diameter

Who Was Excluded: Patients with anatomic factors such as ureteral pelvic junction obstruction, a caliceal diverticulum, or infundibular stenosis. Also excluded were patients with relative contraindications to either approach due to body size or body habitus, coagulopathy, or renal disease (serum creatinine greater than 3 mg/dl).

Patients: 160

Study Overview:
Prospective, randomized, multicenter clinical trial

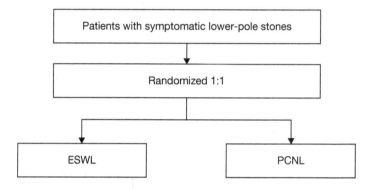

Study Interventions: ESWL versus PCNL and stone retrieval or intracorporeal lithotripsy. The particular ESWL device and the power settings varied by institution, as did the decision to place a stent, though general guidance was given to stent for an aggregate stone size of 25 mm or greater and not to stent for an aggregate diameter of less than 15 mm.

For PCNL, no particular technique of nephrostomy track dilation was specified. Different techniques for stone fragmentation could be applied, such as ultrasound, electrohydraulic fragmentation, and laser.

Follow-Up: Short-term treatment success was assessed at 3 months. The patients were then followed up annually for 3 years thereafter, but the reported results of the study are limited to short-term follow-up.

Endpoints: Primary endpoint: stone-free rate at 3 months. Secondary endpoints: quality-of-life information using the Short Form (SF)-36, blood pressure, and serum creatinine level.

RESULTS:

- Of 160 patients randomized, only 128 ultimately participated. Three-month follow-up for the primary endpoint was available for only 107 patients (66.9%).
- The overall stone-free rates were 37% for ESWL (19/52 cases) and 95% for PCNL (52/55); risk ratio (RR) 0.39 (95% confidence interval [CI], 0.27 to 0.56).
- Rates of retreatment was similar, with 10 patients in each group; RR 1.06 (95% CI, 0.48 to 2.33); auxiliary procedures were required in 5 patients versus 1 patient; RR 5.29 (95% CI, 0.64 to 43.76).
- Hospital stay was longer for the PCNL patients than the ESWL patients (2.66 days [range 1 to 7] vs. 0.55 days [range 0 to 9], respectively, p = 0.0001).
- Complications were less frequent in the SWL group; RR 0.53 (95% CI, 0.21 to 1.31). Complications occurred in 11% and 22% of patients respectively. The complications were mainly minor but tended to be more severe in the PCNL arm.
- Quality-of-life outcomes generally favored ESWL, but none of the differences were statistically significant.

Criticisms and Limitations: The study had a number of methodological limitations, including lack of blinding and a large proportion (more than 30%) of randomized patients not included in the analysis. Stone-related parameters other than location, such as computed tomography (CT)-based Hounsfield unit value and stone-to-skin distance, may influence outcomes of this procedure but were not accounted for.[2] This study only employed single-dimension measurements, which may not represent the true three-dimensional volume of stones.[3,4] More precise and thorough volumetric assessments using imaging software have more recently been introduced. Complication rates reported appear higher than would be expected in contemporary practice.

Other Relevant Studies and Information:

- Ureteroscopy has gained an increasing role for stones of intermediate volume, including lower-pole stones.[6,7]
- Other studies have since used better-defined selection criteria for ESWL patients as a means to obtain higher success rates,[2] and more recent PCNL outcome studies report lower transfusion and morbidity rates.[8]

- Stone studies with CT-based outcome assessment provide more accurate and realistic information about stone-free rates and residual stone burden.[5]
- Two and three dimensions of measurements and more sophisticated volumetric assessments of stone volume are more accurate.[3,4]
- Current evidence-based guidelines by both the American Urological Association and the European Association of Urology recommend against using ESWL in patients with lower-pole renal stones larger than 10 mm.[6,7]

Summary and Implications: This study was the first randomized controlled trial to clarify the tradeoffs of ESWL (low stone clearance rate and frequent need for retreatment, but low morbidity) versus PCNL (high stone-clearance rate and few retreatments, but greater morbidity) for lower-pole renal calculi.

CLINICAL CASE: ESWL VERSUS PCNL FOR LARGE LOWER-POLE CALICEAL STONES

Case History:

An obese 45-year-old male is found to have a 2.5-cm lower-pole stone. He has hypertension and well-controlled diabetes mellitus. He has no history of urinary tract infections. Laboratory testing is normal. Kidney–ureter–bladder (KUB) imaging shows bowel gas and question of a lower-pole density. Non-contrast CT shows a 1.5-cm lower-pole stone with a density of 1,350 Hounsfield units. Stone-to-skin distance is 14.5 cm.

Suggested Answer:

This and subsequent studies would indicate that ESWL is a poor treatment option in this patient based on stone size, density, and stone-to-skin distance. PCNL is indeed effective but is associated with a higher degree of procedure-related morbidity.

References

1. Albala DM, Assimos DG, Clayman RV, et al. Lower pole I: a prospective randomized trial of extracorporeal shock wave lithotripsy and percutaneous nephrostolithotomy for lower pole nephrolithiasis-initial results. *J Urol.* 2001;166(6):2072–80.
2. Elmansy HE, Lingeman JE. Recent advances in lithotripsy technology and treatment strategies: a systematic review update. *Int J Surg.* 2016 Dec;36(Pt D):676–80.

3. Finch W, Johnston R, Shaida N, Winterbottom A, Wiseman O. Measuring stone volume—three-dimensional software reconstruction or an ellipsoid algebra formula? *BJU Int.* 2014 Apr;113(4):610–4.

4. Patel SR, Stanton P, Zelinski N, et al. Automated renal stone volume measurement by noncontrast computerized tomography is more reproducible than manual linear size measurement. *J Urol.* 2011 Dec;186(6):2275–9.

5. Pearle MS, Watamull LM, Mullican MA. Sensitivity of noncontrast helical computerized tomography and plain film radiography compared to flexible nephroscopy for detecting residual fragments after percutaneous nephrostolithotomy. *J Urol.* 1999;162(1):23–6.

6. Assimos D, Krambeck A, Miller NL, et al. Surgical management of stones: American Urological Association/Endourological Society Guideline, part I. *J Urol.* 2016 Oct;196(4):1153–60.

7. Türk C, Petřík A, Sarica K, et al. EAU guidelines on interventional treatment for urolithiasis. *Eur Urol.* 2016 Mar;69(3):475–82.

8. Ghani KR, Andonian S, Bultitude M, et al. Percutaneous nephrolithotomy: update, trends, and future directions. *Eur Urol.* 2016 Aug;70(2):382–96.

37

Medical Expulsive Therapy (MET) in Adults With Ureteric Colic

The Spontaneous Urinary Stone Passage Enabled by Drugs (SUSPEND) Trial

MICHAEL S. BOROFSKY AND VINCENT G. BIRD

"Results of previous studies showed a positive benefit on spontaneous stone passage with [MET]. However, our methodologically sound and large trial offers a strong evidence base for the alternative view that they are unlikely to be useful in the routine clinical care of people with ureteric colic."[1]

Research Question: In patients with ureteral colic, how do alpha-blockers and calcium channel blockers compare to placebo in promoting stone passage and managing symptoms?

Funding: United Kingdom National Institute for Health Research Health Technology Assessment Program

Year Study Began: 2011

Year Study Published: 2015

Study Location: 24 United Kingdom National Health Service hospitals

Who Was Studied: Adults aged 18 to 65 years with one stone of 10 mm or less (in largest dimension) in either ureter identified on computed tomography (CT)

Who Was Excluded: Patients needing immediate intervention, patients with sepsis, patients with an estimated glomerular filtration rate of less than 30 ml/ min, and patients already taking or unable to take an alpha-blocker or calcium channel blocker

Patients: 1,167

Study Overview:

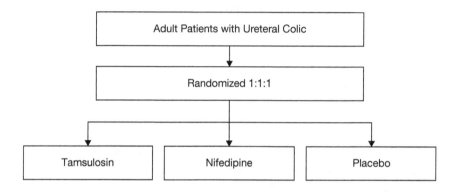

Study Interventions: Participants self-administered tamsulosin 400 µg, nifedipine 30 mg, or placebo orally once daily until spontaneous stone passage occurred, until there was a need for intervention, or until 4 weeks had passed since randomization, whichever came first.

Follow-up: Study duration was 4 weeks, but additional follow-up information was also collected at 12 weeks.

Endpoints: Primary outcome: spontaneous stone passage in 4 weeks, defined as the absence of need for additional interventions. Secondary outcomes: pain, assessed by analgesic use and visual analog scale at 4 weeks; time to stone passage; health status assessed by the Short Form (SF)-36 questionnaire; and discontinuation of medication due to adverse effects and serious adverse events.

RESULTS:

- The mean stone size in all three groups was comparable at 4.5 mm; approximately 75% of stones were 5 mm or less.
- Rates of stone passage (as defined by no need for further intervention) were similar for tamsulosin versus placebo (odds ratio [OR] 1.08; 95% confidence interval [CI], 0.76 to 1.56) and nifedipine versus placebo (OR 1.02; 95% CI, 0.71 to 1.45).
- There was also no difference at 12 weeks, at which time an additional 6% to 7% of participants in each arm required additional interventions.
- There was no indication of subgroup effects based on sex, stone size (5 mm or less vs. more than 5 mm), or stone location (upper, middle, or lower ureter).
- Serious adverse events were very infrequent; there were none in the tamsulosin group, three in the nifedipine group, and one in the placebo group.

Criticism and Limitations: This trial has been criticized for its pragmatic choice of primary outcome as "need for intervention" rather than imaging confirmation of stone passage, ideally by CT.[2-4] There is concern about asymptomatic yet persistent ureteral stone disease causing hydronephrosis and ultimately renal loss.[4] Failure to demonstrate a statistically significant effect may be attributable to a small average stone size with expected high rates of spontaneous passage, leading this study to have been underpowered.

Other Relevant Studies and Information:

- A United States–based study conducted at six emergency departments randomized 512 patients to either tamsulosin or placebo.[5] Mean stone size was 3.8 mm, and follow-up imaging was CT-based. It found similar rates of stone passage between the tamsulosin and placebo groups; RR 1.05 (95% CI, 0.87 to 1.27).
- The largest randomized controlled trial yet, from China, randomized 3,450 patients to tamsulosin versus placebo and included weekly CT imaging for follow-up.[6] It found a 7.8% (95% CI, 5.2% to 10.4%) absolute risk reduction in favor of the tamsulosin group. Subgroup analyses suggested that the observed benefit may mainly derive from patients with larger stones (larger than 5 mm).

- Systematic reviews of over 60 available trials (including SUSPEND) with secondary analyses based on study quality, stone size, and stone location also indicate that the largest benefit is derived in patients with larger stones.[4,7]

Summary and Implications: The SUSPEND trial was a large, methodologically and rigorously conducted trial that failed to demonstrate a benefit from the widely established practice of treating patients with ureteral colic with MET. Based on the totality of evidence, it now appears that MET (e.g., alpha-blockers or calcium channel blockers) may only be beneficial among patients with larger (more than 5 mm) stones.

CLINICAL CASE: MET IN URETERAL COLIC

Case History:
A 35-year-old female presents to the emergency room with a right-sided 3-mm mid-ureteral obstructing stone and pain. She would like to avoid surgery; is there value to prescribing an alpha-blocker to enhance the chance of spontaneous stone passage?

Suggested Answer:
Based on the results of the SUSPEND trial, the likelihood of this patient passing her stone with or without MET is similar. While the addition of MET is unlikely to cause serious adverse effects, the probability that this patient will be able to avoid surgical intervention may not change substantially whether or not she is prescribed MET given her high likelihood (more than 90%) of spontaneous stone passage. Therefore, MET may be omitted, especially if there is heightened concerns about drug side effects. This is consistent with both American Urological Association guidelines that recommend a trial of MET with an alpha-blocker for patients with distal ureteral stones smaller than 10 mm[8] and the European Association of Urology guidelines that recommend a trial of MET with an alpha-blocker for patients with distal ureteral stones larger than 5 mm.[9] Meanwhile, a primary care–based guideline group from the Netherlands, where patients with typical symptoms of ureteral colic are not typically imaged, also recommends the use of alpha-blockers in situations when stone size and location are unknown.[10]

References

1. Pickard R, Starr K, MacLennan G, et al. Medical Expulsive Therapy in Adults with Ureteric Colic: A Multicentre, Randomised, Placebo-Controlled Trial. *Lancet* 2015;386(9991):341–9. doi: 10.1016/S0140-6736(15)60933-3

2. Dahm P, Hollingsworth JM. Medical Expulsive Therapy for Ureteral Stones: Stone Age Medicine. *JAMA Intern Med* 2018;178(8):1058–59. doi: 10.1001/jamainternmed.2018.2265 [published online first: 2018/06/19]

3. Dahm P, Sukumar S, Hollingsworth JM. Medical Expulsive Therapy for Distal Ureteral Stones: The Verdict Is In. *Eur Urol* 2018;73(3):392–3. doi: 10.1016/j.eururo.2017.11.010 [published online first: 2017/11/28]

4. Hollingsworth JM, Canales BK, Rogers MA, et al. Alpha Blockers for Treatment of Ureteric Stones: Systematic Review and Meta-analysis. *BMJ* 2016;355:i6112. doi: 10.1136/bmj.i6112 [published online first: 2016/12/03]

5. Meltzer AC, Burrows PK, Wolfson AB, et al. Effect of Tamsulosin on Passage of Symptomatic Ureteral Stones: A Randomized Clinical Trial. *JAMA Intern Med* 2018;178(8):1051–7. doi: 10.1001/jamainternmed.2018.2259 [published online first: 2018/06/19]

6. Ye Z, Zeng G, Yang H, et al. Efficacy and Safety of Tamsulosin in Medical Expulsive Therapy for Distal Ureteral Stones with Renal Colic: A Multicenter, Randomized, Double-blind, Placebo-Controlled Trial. *Eur Urol* 2018;73(3):385–91. doi: 10.1016/j.eururo.2017.10.033 [published online first: 2017/11/16]

7. Campschroer T, Zhu X, Vernooij RW, et al. Alpha-Blockers as Medical Expulsive Therapy for Ureteral Stones. *Cochrane Database Syst Rev* 2018;4:CD008509. doi: 10.1002/14651858.CD008509.pub3 [published online first: 2018/04/06]

8. Assimos D, Krambeck A, Miller NL, et al. Surgical Management of Stones: American Urological Association/Endourological Society Guideline, Part I. *J Urol* 2016;196(4):1153–60. doi: 10.1016/j.juro.2016.05.090 [published online first: 2016/05/31]

9. Turk C, Knoll T, Seitz C, et al. Medical Expulsive Therapy for Ureterolithiasis: The EAU Recommendations in 2016. *Eur Urol* 2017;71(4):504–7. doi: 10.1016/j.eururo.2016.07.024 [published online first: 2016/08/11]

10. Vermandere M, Kuijpers T, Burgers JS, et al. Alpha-Blockers for Uncomplicated Ureteric Stones: A Clinical Practice Guideline. *BJU Int* 2018;122(6):924–31. doi: 10.1111/bju.14457 [published online first: 2018/07/12]

38

Burch Colposuspension Versus Fascial Sling to Reduce Urinary Stress Incontinence

The Stress Incontinence Surgical Treatment Efficacy (SISTEr) Trial

COLBY A. DIXON, GIULIA I. LANE, CYNTHIA S. FOK, AND M. LOUIS MOY

"The autologous fascial sling results in a higher rate of successful treatment of stress incontinence but also greater morbidity than the Burch colposuspension."[1]

Research Question: In women with stress urinary incontinence (SUI), how does an autologous rectus fascial sling compare to a Burch colposuspension procedure?

Funding: National Institute of Diabetes, Digestive and Kidney Diseases (NIDDK), National Institute of Child Health and Human Development (NICHD), Office of Research in Women's Health (ORWH) of the National Institutes of Health (NIH)

Year Study Began: 2002

Year Study Published: 2007

Study Location: Nine clinical centers across the United States as part of the Urinary Incontinence Treatment Network (UITN)

Who Was Studied: Women with stress-predominant urinary incontinence

Who Was Excluded: Women with prior pelvic surgery or radiation or those who were pregnant

Patients: 655

Study Overview:

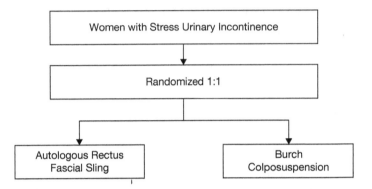

Study Interventions: Women in the intervention arm underwent an autologous rectus fascial sling procedure, those in the control arm a Burch colposuspension. The key elements of each surgical procedure were standardized across all surgeons; concomitant prolapse repairs were permitted. Patients were informed postoperatively which procedure they had undergone. Follow-up was in the format of interviews and clinical exams conducted at 6 weeks and at 3, 6, 12, 18, and 24 months postoperatively.

Follow-up: 24 months

Endpoints: Primary outcomes: overall treatment success (negative pad test, no self-reported leakage on 3-day voiding diary, no self-reported SUI symptoms, negative stress test, no retreatment) and SUI-specific treatment success (negative stress test, no self-reported SUI symptoms, no retreatment). Secondary outcomes: complications, quality of life, sexual function, treatment expectations, patient satisfaction.

RESULTS:

- Overall treatment success favored the fascial sling over the Burch procedure group (47% vs. 38%, p = 0.01) as did the SUI-specific success rate (66% vs. 49%, p < 0.001) at 24 months.
- Rates of serious adverse events were similar, but minor adverse events (e.g., urinary tract infections) were more common in the sling group (63% vs. 47%, p < 0.001).
- Postoperative voiding dysfunction (14% vs. 2%, p < 0.001) and urge incontinence (27% vs. 20%, p = 0.04) were more common in the sling group than the Burch group.
- Treatment satisfaction at 24 months was higher in the sling group than the Burch group (86% vs. 78%, p = 0.02).
- There was no apparent effect of concomitant prolapse surgery on outcome measures in either group.

Criticism and Limitations: The study used a multicomponent composite outcome that included endpoints of different degrees of patient importance and frequency.[2] A secondary analysis also found that only about a third of patients completed all four measures (Medical, Epidemiologic and Social Aspects of Aging [MESA] stress index, voiding diary, stress test, pad test) that defined the primary outcome measures.[3] Whereas urinary tract infection rates favored the Burch approach, it was based on clinical suspicion rather than culture confirmation. Today the study's applicability has been limited by the widespread use of synthetic (rather than autologous) midurethral slings.

Other Relevant Studies and Information:

- The investigators have reported a 5-year extension of the trial in which three-quarters (482 of 655) of patients participated.[4] At 5 years, continence rates remained higher in the sling group than in the Burch group (31% vs. 24%, p = 0.002). Satisfaction was also higher in the sling group (83% vs. 73%, p = 0.04), although overall satisfaction decreased over time in both groups. There was no significant difference in long-term rates of adverse events.
- A Cochrane review has found low-quality evidence overall that women may be more likely to be continent in the medium term (1

to 5 years) after a traditional suburethral sling operation than after colposuspension.[5]

Summary and Implications: In this head-to-head comparison, patients who underwent sling placement had better continence outcomes than those who underwent colposuspension. There were, however, higher rates of urinary tract infection, voiding dysfunction, and urge incontinence among those receiving sling placement. These findings have supported a shift toward slings (autologous and synthetic) versus Burch colposuspension procedures in clinical practice.

CLINICAL CASE: AUTOLOGOUS FASCIA PUBOVAGINAL SLING VERSUS BURCH COLPOSUSPENSION

Case History:
An otherwise healthy 42-year-old woman presents to your office desiring surgical management for a 3-year history of refractory SUI. Her physical examination is remarkable for observation of leakage with cough and Valsalva and urethral hypermobility. There is no concomitant vaginal prolapse. Given considerable controversy around mesh-related complications[6,7] that have led to its restricted use in the United Kingdom, Australia, and New Zealand,[8] she is adamant that no synthetic mesh be used. What can you offer her?

Suggested Answer:
The patient strongly opposes a synthetic midurethral sling, which current guidelines by the European Association of Urology regard as the first choice in patients with uncomplicated SUI like her.[9] Meanwhile, guidelines of the American Urological Association list synthetic midurethral slings, autologous fascia pubovaginal slings, and Burch colposuspension all as first-line approaches with specific advantages and disadvantages.[10] Based on the SISTEr trial, an autologous fascia pubovaginal sling would be favored with regard to better incontinence outcomes. However, the added morbidity of the fascial harvest should be discussed with her.

References

1. Brubaker L, Cundiff GW, Fine P, et al. Abdominal sacrocolpopexy with Burch colposuspension to reduce urinary stress incontinence. *N Engl J Med* 2006;354(15):1557–66. doi: 10.1056/NEJMoa054208 [published online first: 2006/04/14]

2. Montori VM, Permanyer-Miralda G, Ferreira-Gonzalez I, et al. Validity of composite end points in clinical trials. *BMJ* 2005;330(7491):594–6.

3. Brubaker L, Litman HJ, Kim HY, et al. Missing data frequency and correlates in two randomized surgical trials for urinary incontinence in women. *Int Urogynecol J* 2015;26(8):1155–9. doi: 10.1007/s00192-015-2661-5 [published online first: 2015/03/25]

4. Brubaker L, Richter HE, Norton PA, et al. 5-year continence rates, satisfaction and adverse events of Burch urethropexy and fascial sling surgery for urinary incontinence. *J Urol* 2012;187(4):1324–30. doi: 10.1016/j.juro.2011.11.087 [published online first: 2012/02/22]

5. Saraswat L, Rehman H, Omar MI, et al. Traditional suburethral sling operations for urinary incontinence in women. *Cochrane Database Syst Rev* 2020;1:CD001754. doi: 10.1002/14651858.CD001754.pub5 [published online first: 2020/01/29]

6. Gurol-Urganci I, Geary RS, Mamza JB, et al. Long-term rate of mesh sling removal following midurethral mesh sling insertion among women with stress urinary incontinence. *JAMA* 2018;320(16):1659–69. doi: 10.1001/jama.2018.14997 [published online first: 2018/10/26]

7. Heneghan C, Godlee F. Surgical mesh and patient safety. *BMJ* 2018;363:k4231. doi: 10.1136/bmj.k4231 [published online first: 2018/10/12]

8. Hofner K, Hampel C, Kirschner-Hermanns R, et al. [Use of synthetic slings and mesh implants in the treatment of female stress urinary incontinence and prolapse: Statement of the Working Group on Urological Functional Diagnostics and Female Urology of the Academy of the German Society of Urology]. *Urologe A* 2020;59(1):65–71. doi: 10.1007/s00120-019-01074-y [published online first: 2019/11/20]

9. Burkhard FC, Bosch JLHR, Cruz F, et al. Urinary incontinence: European Association of Urology; 2020 [EAU guideline]. Available from: https://uroweb.org/guideline/urinary-incontinence/#note_308. Accessed 1/30/2020.

10. Kobashi KC, Albo M, Dmochowski RR, et al. Surgical treatment of female stress urinary incontinence (SUI): AUA/SUFU guideline (2017): American Urological Association; 2017. Available from: https://www.auanet.org/guidelines/stress-urinary-incontinence-(sui)-guideline. Accessed 1/30/2020.

39

Retropubic Versus Transobturator Midurethral Slings for Stress Incontinence

The Trial of Mid Urethral Slings (TOMUS)

GIULIA I. LANE, COLBY A. DIXON, M. LOUIS MOY, AND
CYNTHIA S. FOK

"This large, multicenter, comparative-effectiveness trial showed that there was statistical and clinical equivalence in the rates of treatment success according to objective criteria between the two most commonly performed midurethral sling procedures for the treatment of stress incontinence in women."[1]

Research Question: In women with stress urinary incontinence (SUI), how do retropubic midurethral slings versus transobturator slings compare?

Funding: National Institute of Diabetes and Digestive and Kidney Diseases and National Institute of Child Health and Human Development

Year Study Began: 2006

Year Study Published: 2010

Study Location: Nine tertiary care centers in the United States that constitute the Urinary Incontinence Treatment Network (UITN)[2]

Who Was Studied: Women 21 years and older with predominantly stress-type urinary incontinence

Who Was Excluded: Pregnant women and those within 12 months of delivery, women with history of any incontinence surgery

Patients: 583

Study Overview:

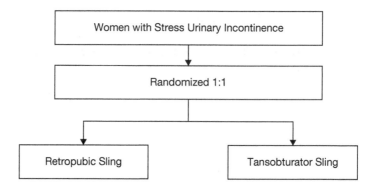

Study Interventions: Women in the retropubic arm underwent a Tension-free Vaginal Tape (Gynecare). Women in the transobturator sling underwent a Tension-free Vaginal Tape Obturator (Gynecare) performed via an "in-to-out" approach or the Monarc (American Medical Systems) performed via an "out-to-in" approach. Patients were followed at 2 weeks, 6 weeks, 6 months, and 12 months postoperatively with questionnaires, clinical interviews, and exams. The study was designed as an equivalence study

Follow-up: 12 months

Endpoints: Primary outcome: composite consisting of an objective and subjective component. The objective criteria were a negative provocative urinary stress test, a negative 24-hour pad test, and no retreatment for SUI. The subjective criteria were absence of self-reported symptoms of SUI based on the Medical, Epidemiological, and Social Aspects of Aging (MESA) questionnaire, no leakage recorded in a 3-day voiding diary, and no retreatment for SUI. The study was designed as an equivalence study with two-sided 12% equivalence margins based on a per-protocol analysis.

RESULTS:

- The mean patient age was approximately 53 years, and approximately 80% were non-Hispanic white.
- The median baseline pad weight was approximately 12 grams and the median number of incontinence episodes was 2.7.
- At 12 months 80.8% of the retropubic group and 77.7% of the transobturator group met the criteria for objective treatment success; absolute risk difference: +3.0 (95% confidence interval [CI], −3.6 to +9.6), consistent with equivalence.
- Subjective treatment success criteria were met by 62.2% of the retropubic group and 55.8% of the transobturator group; absolute risk difference: +6.4 (95% CI, −1.6 to +14.3), favoring the retropubic approach.
- Study outcomes were not sensitive to secondary analyses by clinical site, Valsalva leak point pressure, or maximal urethral closure pressure.
- The retropubic sling group had more serious adverse events than the transobturator sling group (43 vs. 20 events, respectively; p = 0.003).
- Bladder perforations and voiding dysfunction only occurred in the retropubic sling group; neurologic symptoms (weakness and numbness) were significantly more common in the transobturator group than the retropubic group (31 vs. 15 events, p = 0.01).

Criticism and Limitations: This was an open-label study with a short-term follow-up of 12 months. Its composite endpoint combined a variety of endpoints of differing patient importance. The predetermined margins for equivalence of 12% in both directions were quite wide.

Other Relevant Studies and Information:

- Extended follow-up outcomes at 2 years and 5 years indicate decreasing success rates for both approaches but continued to favor the retropubic arm.[3,4]
- A Cochrane review identified 55 randomized controlled trials comparing retropubic versus transobturator slings and found similar outcomes in terms of symptomatic improvement and cure rates at 12 months, 12 months to 5 years, and more than 5 years.[5]

Summary and Implications: Based on this and subsequent studies, retropubic and transobturator midurethral sling approaches appear to have equivalent outcomes at 12 months for the treatment of SUI. However, the approaches differ in their adverse event profiles and patients should be counseled on the unique risks associated with each procedure.

CLINICAL CASE: RETROPUBIC VERSUS TRANSOBTURATOR MIDURETHRAL SLING

Case History:

A 52-year-old, otherwise healthy female presents with a 1-year history of purely SUI. Clinical exam demonstrates a positive urinary stress test at bladder volume of 150 cc. After discussion about potential management approaches, the patient elects for midurethral sling to treat her SUI. How would you counsel this patient with regard to retropubic versus transobturator sling?

Suggested Answer:

Both the American Urological Association and the European Association of Urology (EAU) state that both approaches are appropriate, with EAU guidelines indicating that midurethral synthetic slings inserted by the retropubic route have higher objective long-term (8 years) patient-reported cure rates.[6,7] The retropubic route of insertion is associated with a higher intraoperative risk of bladder perforation and a higher rate of voiding dysfunction than the transobturator route; the transobturator route of insertion is associated with a higher risk of groin pain than the retropubic route. Based on this informed discussion, the patient elects a retropubic approach.

References

1. Richter HE, Albo ME, Zyczynski HM, et al. Retropubic versus transobturator midurethral slings for stress incontinence. *N Engl J Med* 2010;362(22):2066–76. doi: 10.1056/NEJMoa0912658

2. Urinary Incontinence Treatment Network. The Trial of Mid-Urethral Slings (TOMUS): design and methodology. *J Appl Res* 2008;8(1):AlboVol8No1 [published online first: 2008/01/01]

3. Albo ME, Litman HJ, Richter HE, et al. Treatment success of retropubic and transobturator mid urethral slings at 24 months. *J Urol* 2012;188(6):2281–7. doi: 10.1016/j.juro.2012.07.103 [published online first: 2012/10/23]

4. Kenton K, Stoddard AM, Zyczynski H, et al. 5-year longitudinal followup after retropubic and transobturator mid urethral slings. *J Urol* 2015;193(1):203–10. doi: 10.1016/j.juro.2014.08.089 [published online first: 2014/08/27]

5. Ford AA, Rogerson L, Cody JD, et al. Mid-urethral sling operations for stress urinary incontinence in women. *Cochrane Database Syst Rev* 2017;7:CD006375. doi: 10.1002/14651858.CD006375.pub4 [published online first: 2017/08/02]

6. Burkhard FC, Bosch JLHR, Cruz F, et al. Urinary incontinence: European Association of Urology; 2020 [EAU guideline]. Available from: https://uroweb. org/guideline/urinary-incontinence/#note_308. Accessed 1/30/2020.

7. Kobashi KC, Albo M, Dmochowski RR, et al. Surgical treatment of female stress urinary incontinence (SUI): AUA/SUFU Guideline (2017): American Urological Association; 2017. Available from: https://www.auanet.org/guidelines/stress-urinary-incontinence-(sui)-guideline. Accessed 1/30/2020.

40

A Midurethral Sling to Reduce Incontinence After Vaginal Prolapse Repair

The Outcomes Following Vaginal Prolapse Repair and Midurethral Sling (OPUS) Trial

GIULIA I. LANE, COLBY A. DIXON, M. LOUIS MOY, AND CYNTHIA S. FOK

"A prophylactic midurethral sling inserted during vaginal prolapse surgery resulted in a lower rate of urinary incontinence at 3 and 12 months but higher rates of adverse events."[1]

Research Question: In women without stress urinary incontinence (SUI) undergoing prolapse surgery, how do incontinence symptoms compare with or without concomitant midurethral sling (MUS)?

Funding: Office of Research on Women's Health; National Institute of Diabetes and Digestive and Kidney Diseases; Eunice Kennedy Shriver National Institute of Child Health and Human Development

Year Study Began: 2007

Year Study Published: 2012

Study Location: Multicenter study recruiting from tertiary care centers in the United States that constituted the Pelvic Floor Disorders Network (PFDN)[2]

Who Was Studied: Women with stage 2 or higher pelvic organ prolapse (as defined by the Pelvic Organ Prolapse Quantification system) scheduled to undergo vaginal prolapse surgery without SUI

Who Was Excluded: Women with a history of prior MUS placement, women currently receiving treatment for SUI, women with contraindications to MUS, women planning a pregnancy within 1 year after surgery, women with a history of two or more hospitalizations within the prior year for medical illness

Patients: 337

Study Overview:

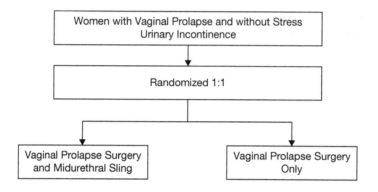

Study Interventions: Women in the intervention group underwent vaginal prolapse surgery and a retropubic MUS using the Gynecare tension-free vaginal tape (TVT, Ethicon). Women in the control group underwent vaginal prolapse surgery as well as two additional superficial sham incisions above the pubic bone.

Follow-up: 12 months

Endpoints: Co-primary endpoints were a composite of stress, urge, or mixed urinary incontinence (UI) as defined by a positive cough stress test, bothersome UI symptoms, or treatment for UI at 3 months and 12 months. Secondary outcomes included bladder symptoms, pelvic organ prolapse, adverse events, and health-related quality-of-life data as assessed by validated patient questionnaires at 3, 6, and 12 months of follow-up.

RESULTS:

- Rates of UI at 3 months were 23.6% in the sling group versus 49.4% in the sham group. Women in the sling group had lower rates of positive cough stress test and bothersome symptoms but had similar rates of postoperative treatment of UI. The number needed to treat to prevent one case of UI at 3 months was 4.
- Rates of UI at 12 months were 27.3% in the sling group versus 43.0% in the sham group. The difference in patient-reported symptoms of UI between the sling group (11.4%) versus the sham group (18.8%) was not statistically significant (p = 0.07).
- At 12 months, 7.3% of patients in the sling group and 11% in the sham group underwent subsequent treatment for UI. The number needed to treat to prevent one case of UI at 12 months was 7.
- At 3 months, the sling group had greater improvement from baseline on the Pelvic Floor Distress Inventory (PFDI) and Incontinence Severity Index, but the PFDI results were not durable to 12 months.
- Bladder perforation (6.7% vs. 0%), urinary tract infection (31.0% vs. 18.3%), major bleeding complications (3.1% vs. 0.0%), and incomplete bladder emptying after 6 weeks (3.7% vs. 0.0%) were all more common in the sling group.

Criticism and Limitations: The type of vaginal surgery for pelvic organ pro-lapse performed was heterogeneous and the study was not designed to explore associations between the type of prolapse surgery and rates of UI. Follow-up was limited to 12 months.

Other Relevant Studies and Information:

- Findings of this study support those of the Colpopexy and Urinary Reduction Efforts (CARE) trial, which randomized patients to concomitant Burch colposuspension or no Burch colposuspension at the time of abdominal sacrocolpopexy for apical prolapse.[3]
- Based on an observational study from the Netherlands, continence rates at 24 months are similar to those at 12 months in patients undergoing TVT with and without concomitant surgery.[4]
- The PFDN developed a validated model for predicting de novo SUI based on the data from the OPUS trial.[5]

• A systematic review that included up to seven trials of prolapse surgery with or without various forms of SUI surgery also supports a reduced rate of de novo SUI but an increased rate of adverse events.[6]

Summary and Implications: The OPUS trial found that women randomized to undergo prophylactic concomitant MUS at the time of transvaginal repair for pelvic organ prolapse had lower rates of UI at 3 and 12 months but higher rates of adverse events. These findings offer important data to inform the decision regarding whether or not to perform a concomitant MUS at the time of transvaginal pelvic organ prolapse repair.

CLINICAL CASE: PROPHYLACTIC SLING SURGERY AT THE TIME OF VAGINAL PROLAPSE REPAIR

Case History:
A 63-year-old female presents with a bothersome vaginal bulge with no UI symptoms. Physical exam shows that the vaginal wall is 1.5 cm below the hymenal ring, and with the prolapse reduced, cough stress test with 200 ml is negative. The patient is nervous about undergoing surgery but ultimately elects for transvaginal repair of her prolapse. How would you counsel this patient regarding MUS at the time of prolapse repair?

Suggested Answer:
The OPUS trial suggests that as many as one in two women may develop some degree of UI following prolapse repair. This risk can be reduced through prophylactic, concomitant placement of a sling, but side effects are also substantially increased. The alternative would be secondary surgical treatment of the de novo UI in patients who have failed conservative management. Current evidence-based guidelines by the National Institute for Health and Care Excellence (NICE) recommend that surgical candidates be counseled that there is a risk of developing postoperative UI and further treatment may be needed but not to offer them prophylactic surgery.[7] Assuming that the patient is accepting of her risk of de novo UI and prefers to minimize her surgical interventions, vaginal prolapse surgery alone appears the most appropriate approach.

References

1. Wei JT, Nygaard I, Richter HE, et al. A midurethral sling to reduce incontinence after vaginal prolapse repair. *N Engl J Med* 2012;366(25):2358–67. doi: 10.1056/ NEJMoa1111967

2. Wei J, Nygaard I, Richter H, et al. Outcomes following vaginal prolapse repair and midurethral sling (OPUS) trial: design and methods. *Clin Trials* 2009;6(2):162–71. doi: 10.1177/1740774509102605 [published online first: 2009/04/04]

3. Brubaker L, Cundiff GW, Fine P, et al. Abdominal sacrocolpopexy with Burch colposuspension to reduce urinary stress incontinence. *N Engl J Med* 2006;354(15):1557–66. doi: 10.1056/NEJMoa054208 [published online first: 2006/04/14]

4. Schraffordt Koops SE, Bisseling TM, van Brummen HJ, et al. Result of the tension-free vaginal tape in patients with concomitant prolapse surgery: a 2-year follow-up study. An analysis from the Netherlands TVT database. *Int Urogynecol J Pelvic Floor Dysfunct* 2007;18(4):437–42. doi: 10.1007/s00192-006-0170-2 [published online first: 2006/08/16]

5. Jelovsek JE, Chagin K, Brubaker L, et al. A model for predicting the risk of de novo stress urinary incontinence in women undergoing pelvic organ prolapse surgery. *Obstet Gynecol* 2014;123(2 Pt 1):279–87. doi: 10.1097/AOG.0000000000000094 [published online first: 2014/01/10]

6. van der Ploeg JM, van der Steen A, Oude Rengerink K, et al. Prolapse surgery with or without stress incontinence surgery for pelvic organ prolapse: a systematic review and meta-analysis of randomised trials. *Br J Obstet Gynaecol* 2014;121(5):537–47. doi: 10.1111/1471-0528.12509 [published online first: 2014/01/03]

7. NICE. Guidance—Urinary incontinence and pelvic organ prolapse in women: management. *BJU Int* 2019;123(5):777–803. doi: 10.1111/bju.14763 [published online first: 2019/04/23]

41

A Randomized Trial of Urodynamic Testing Before Stress Incontinence Surgery

The Value of Urodynamic Evaluation (ValUE) Trial

COLBY A. DIXON, GIULIA I. LANE, CYNTHIA S. FOK, AND M. LOUIS MOY

"For women with uncomplicated, demonstrable stress urinary incontinence, preoperative office evaluation alone was not inferior to evaluation with urodynamic testing for outcomes at 1 year."[1]

Research Question: In women with stress urinary incontinence (SUI) scheduled to undergo surgery, do outcomes differ in patients undergoing preoperative urodynamic studies (UDS) versus office evaluation only?

Funding: National Institute of Diabetes and Digestive and Kidney Diseases and Eunice Kennedy Shriver National Institute of Child Health and Human Development

Year Study Began: 2008

Year Study Published: 2012

Study Location: 11 clinical centers across the United States as part of the Urinary Incontinence Treatment Network (UITN)

Who Was Studied: Women with uncomplicated, stress-predominant urinary incontinence who were planning to undergo surgery

Who Was Excluded: Women who had previous surgery for incontinence, pelvic radiation, recent pelvic surgery, and anterior or apical prolapse greater than 1 cm distal to the hymenal ring

Patients: 630

Study Overview:

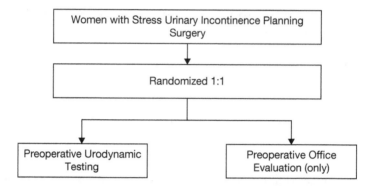

Study Interventions: Women in the intervention arm underwent UDS, which consisted of a noninvasive uroflow, filling cytometry with Valsalva leak point pressures, and pressure flow study, in addition to standard office evaluation. Women in the control group only had a standard office evaluation that consisted of performing a stress test, postvoid residual, assessment of urethral hypermobility, and testing for bladder infection. Patients then underwent SUI surgery with one of six procedures based on surgeon preference. Outcome data were obtained at office visits 3 months and 12 months postoperatively. The study was designed as a non-inferiority study with an 11-point margin.

Follow-up: 12 months

Endpoints: Primary outcome: overall treatment success at 12 months as defined by two validated instruments (reduction of at least 70% in the score on the Urogenital Distress Inventory and a response of "much better" or "very much better" on the Patient Global Impression of Improvement). Secondary outcomes: incontinence severity, quality of life, patient satisfaction, rates of positive provocative stress test, adverse events.

RESULTS:

- Treatment was considered successful at 12 months in 76.9% of the UDS group versus 77.2% of the evaluation-only group.
- A primary diagnosis of SUI was confirmed in 97% of the patients who underwent UDS.
- Of the 315 patients who underwent UDS, changes in the planned surgical approach were made for 18 patients based on UDS results.
- There were no significant differences between the groups for secondary outcome measures including disease severity, quality of life, positive provocative stress test, adverse events, and patient satisfaction.
- Women who underwent preoperative UDS were more likely to be given a diagnosis of voiding phase dysfunction and were less likely to be given a diagnosis of overactive bladder, but this did not result in a change in distribution of overall surgical treatment.

Criticism and Limitations: First, there were imbalances between the two study groups for important variables such as duration and severity of symptoms, prior incontinence treatment, estrogen therapy, and urethral hypermobility, which may have favored the non-inferiority conclusion. Second, patients were treated with six different types of surgical intervention with different outcome profiles[2] that might have obscured the potential value of UDS. Follow-up of the trial was short at 12 months and the non-inferiority margin was wide. Study findings are not applicable to women with complicating factors such as mixed incontinence, concomitant prolapse, prior surgery, or neurologic disease.[1]

Other Relevant Studies and Information:

- A similar yet smaller non-inferiority study randomized patients in whom there was a discordance between office evaluations and UDS findings to a midurethral sling surgery versus tailored treatment based on UDS findings. The mean improvement in symptoms at 1 year was higher in the group who underwent immediate surgery, also supporting little added value of preoperative UDS.[3]
- Currently the joint American Urologic Association/Society of Urodynamics, Female Pelvic Medicine and Urogenital Reconstruction (AUA/SUFU) guideline[4] on female SUI state that physicians may omit UDS for the index patient when SUI is clearly demonstrated and may perform UDS in non-index patients. Similarly, the European

Association of Urology (EAU) guidelines[5] state that performing preoperative UDS in women with uncomplicated, clinically demonstrable SUI does not improve the outcome of surgery for SUI; they do not recommend routinely performing UDS prior to treating uncomplicated SUI.

Summary and Implications: These findings suggest that UDS may not contribute to the overall success rate of surgery in healthy women with uncomplicated SUI. These findings are not applicable to patients with mixed incontinence or other complicating factors, however.

CLINICAL CASE: PREOPERATIVE EVALUATION PRIOR TO MIDURETHRAL SLING SURGERY

Case History:

A healthy 43-year-old woman presents to your office desiring surgical treatment for a 3-year history of urinary incontinence with coughing, sneezing, and lifting. She has had no prior pelvic surgeries, no known neurologic disease, nor any urinary complaints. What is the appropriate preoperative workup for this patient?

Suggested Answer:

This woman matches the index patient for uncomplicated SUI for both the AUA/SUFU and EAU guidelines.[4,5] Her initial office evaluation should consist of a thorough history including details of the type, timing, and severity of symptoms as well as general medical and surgical history. A physician history may be supplemented by one of multiple validated questionnaires to allow for differentiation between stress, urgency, and mixed incontinence. Voiding diaries may also be useful in quantifying symptoms and are recommended but not mandated by either guideline. A focused physical exam should also be performed, including a pelvic exam to assess for concomitant prolapse, fistula, or other genitourinary abnormality. The patient should be asked to cough or strain with a comfortably full bladder and objective visualization of leak should be attempted. The AUA and EAU also recommend assessment of postvoid residual to rule out urinary retention and urinalysis (and urine culture if indicated) to assess for bladder infection. If the results of this initial workup confirm uncomplicated SUI, patients may proceed directly to a midurethral sling without undergoing UDS or other additional testing. Whereas National

Institute for Health and Care Excellence (NICE) guidelines do not recommend midurethral slings, they also state that there is no role for UDS in women with uncomplicated SUI.[6]

References

1. Nager CW, Brubaker L, Litman HJ, et al. A randomized trial of urodynamic testing before stress-incontinence surgery. *N Engl J Med.* 2012;366(21):1987–1997.
2. Imamura M, Hudson J, Wallace SA, et al. Surgical interventions for women with stress urinary incontinence: systematic review and network meta-analysis of randomised controlled trials. *BMJ.* 2019;365:l1842.
3. van Leijsen SA, Kluivers KB, Mol BW, et al. Value of urodynamics before stress urinary incontinence surgery: a randomized controlled trial. *Obstet Gynecol.* 2013;121(5):999–1008.
4. Kobashi KC, Albo M, Dmochowski RR, et al. Surgical treatment of female stress urinary incontinence (SUI): AUA/SUFU guideline (2017): American Urological Association; 2017. Available from: https://www.auanet.org/guidelines/stress-urinary-incontinence-(sui)-guideline. Accessed 1/30/2020.
5. Burkhard FC, Bosch JLHR, Cruz F, et al. Urinary incontinence: European Association of Urology; 2020 [EAU Guideline]. Available from: https://uroweb.org/guideline/urinary-incontinence/#note_308. Accessed 1/30/2020.
6. NICE. Guidance—urinary incontinence and pelvic organ prolapse in women: management. *BJU Int* 2019;123(5):777–803. doi: 10.1111/bju.14763 [published online first: 2019/04/23]

42

Anticholinergic Therapy Versus Onabotulinumtoxin A for Urgency Urinary Incontinence

The Anticholinergic Versus Botulinum Toxin Comparison (ABC) Study

GIULIA I. LANE, COLBY A. DIXON, M. LOUIS MOY, AND CYNTHIA S. FOK

"In summary, we found that among women with urgency urinary incontinence, there was no significant difference between anticholinergic drugs and onabotulinumtoxin A by injection on the reduction of the frequency of episodes of urgency incontinence or improvements in quality of life."[1]

Research Question: In women with urgency urinary incontinence (UUI), how does daily oral anticholinergic therapy compare to a one-time intradetrusor injection of 100 units onabotulinumtoxin A (Botox) with respect to episodes of incontinence?

Funding: Funded by the Eunice Kennedy Shriver National Institute of Child Health and Human Development, National Institutes of Health Office of Research on Women's Health

Year Study Began: 2010

Year Study Published: 2012

Study Location: Multicenter study at 10 centers in the United States

Who Was Studied: Women at least 21 years of age with at least five UUI episodes on a 3-day voiding diary and urge-predominant incontinence who requested treatment for UUI

Who Was Excluded: Women unable to perform intermittent catheterization; women who had prior treatment with or contraindications to the trial agents; women with prior pelvic floor or bladder pathologies or surgery, and prior neuromodulation or neurologic disorders[1]

Patients: 249

Study Overview:

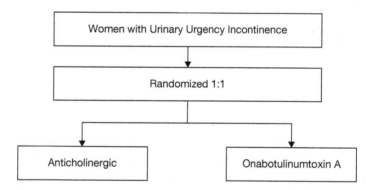

Study Interventions: Women in the anticholinergic arm received solifenacin 5 mg daily and one cystoscopy with intradetrusor injection of saline. The Botox group received daily oral placebo and one cystoscopy with intradetrusor injections of a total of 100 units Botox.

Follow-up: 6 months (followed by open-label extension up to 12 months)

Endpoints: Primary outcome: change in the mean number of UUI episodes over the course of 6 months, as reported for 3-day periods in monthly bladder diaries, compared to baseline. Secondary outcomes: proportion of participants with complete resolution of UUI; proportion with more than 75% reduction in UUI; scores on several validated quality-of-life questionnaires; and adverse events.

RESULTS:

- The baseline mean episodes of UUI was 5.2 ± 2.7 in the anticholinergic group and 4.8 ± 2.7 in the Botox group.
- The reported change in the mean number of UUI episodes between the two interventions was similar (reduction of 3.4 episodes per day in the anticholinergic group and 3.3 in the Botox group, p = 0.81).
- In preplanned subgroup analyses, the treatment effect did not differ by prior anticholinergic treatment or not or baseline frequency of urgency incontinence.
- Complete resolution of symptoms was more likely in the Botox group (27% vs. 13%, p = 0.003).
- Both groups showed improved quality of life without significant differences between interventions based on validated questionnaires.
- At 6 months, there was no difference in the percentage of patients who reported adequate control of symptoms (71% anticholinergic vs. 70% Botox).
- Rates of serious adverse events (5% vs. 3%) and any adverse events (69% vs. 73%) were similar for the anticholinergic group versus the Botox group, respectively.
- A dry mouth was reported more frequently by women in the anticholinergic group (46% vs. 31%); women in the Botox group had higher rates of urinary tract infections (33% vs. 13%).
- More women in the Botox group reported self-catherization, especially early on after the injection.

Criticism and Limitations: The study lacked a sham/placebo group to assess the incremental benefit of either treatment modality. Blinded follow-up was relatively short at 6 months, reflecting the time-limited effect of Botox injections into the bladder.

Other Relevant Studies and Information:

- A cost-effectiveness analysis that was published based on the ABC trial found that there were no differences in total direct and indirect costs at 6 months between the two treatment approaches. At 9 months, assuming no repeat Botox treatment, the total direct cost of Botox was significantly lower than anticholinergic ($1,266 vs. $1,942, p < 0.01).[2]

- A Cochrane review found Botox injection to be an effective treatment for refractory overactive bladder symptoms.[3]

Summary and Implications: The ABC study remains the only randomized controlled trial of Botox injection versus anticholinergic therapy. It demonstrated similar outcomes for both treatments with respect to symptoms of urinary incontinence. Botox injections were associated with more urinary tract infections and higher rates of patients requiring intermittent catherization. Based on these findings, major guidelines indicate that Botox bladder injections should be a third-line therapy (alongside peripheral and tibial nerve stimulation) in patients who have failed behavioral modification and initial pharmacological therapy.[4,5]

CLINICAL CASE: ANTICHOLINERGIC THERAPY VERSUS BOTOX FOR UUI

Case History:

A 58-year-old woman presents with symptoms of pure UUI. She completes a 3-day voiding diary with findings of four UUI episodes per day. She lives an active lifestyle that she is unwilling to change and is quite bothered by these symptoms. She has tried a number of anticholinergic medications but found the side effects (dry mouth, constipation) very disagreeable. She has no prior surgical or medical history. Physical exam shows no pelvic organ prolapse and no leakage on cough stress test. How can you best counsel this patient on management options?

Suggested Answer:

Current evidence-based guidelines recommend a stepwise approach to the management of overactive bladder progressing from behavioral therapy to pharmacological therapy and then surgical interventions.[4,5] This patient has failed to respond to behavioral modification and several medications such as solifenacin and trospium XR, making Botox bladder injections a suitable option; other drugs are likely to have similar side effects. Based on this trial, she can be informed that the average patient can expect a reduction of three UUI episodes per day. However, she will be at a higher risk for urinary retention and urinary tract infections following the procedure.

References

1. Visco AG, Brubaker L, Richter HE, et al. Anticholinergic therapy vs. onabotulinumtoxin A for urgency urinary incontinence. *N Engl J Med.* 2012;367(19):1803–13.

2. Visco AG, Zyczynski H, Brubaker L, et al. Cost-effectiveness analysis of anticholinergics versus Botox for urgency urinary incontinence: results from the Anticholinergic Versus Botox Comparison randomized trial. *Female Pelvic Med Reconstr Surg.* 2016;22(5):311–6.

3. Duthie JB, Vincent M, Herbison GP, et al. Botulinum toxin injections for adults with overactive bladder syndrome. *Cochrane Database Syst Rev.* 2011(12):CD005493.

4. Gormley EA, Lightner DJ, Burgio KL, et al. Diagnosis and treatment of overactive bladder (non-neurogenic) in adults: AUA/SUFU guideline. *J Urol.* 2012;188(6 Suppl):2455–63.

5. Lucas MG, Bosch RJ, Burkhard FC, et al. EAU guidelines on surgical treatment of urinary incontinence. *Eur Urol.* 2012;62(6):1118–29.

Oral Sildenafil in the Treatment of Erectile Dysfunction

JOSHUA BODIE

"Oral sildenafil is an effective, well tolerated treatment for men with erectile dysfunction."[1]

Research Question: In men with erectile dysfunction (ED), how do different doses of oral sildenafil compare to placebo?

Funding: Pfizer

Year Study Began: Not reported

Year Study Published: 1998

Study Location: 37 medical centers in the United States

Who Was Studied: Men ages 18 and older with a clinical diagnosis of ED of organic, psychogenic, or mixed etiology

Who Was Excluded: Men with other penile disorders such as Peyronie's disease, premature ejaculation, spinal cord injury, or other serious medical comorbidities such as poorly controlled diabetes

Patients: 532

Study Overview:

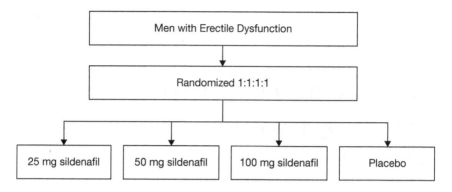

Study Interventions: Patients received either an identical placebo or 25-mg, 50-mg, or 100-mg tablets of sildenafil to be taken approximately 1 hour before planned sexual activity (but not more than once daily) for 24 weeks. Each man completed the International Index of Erectile Function (IIEF) at 0, 12, and 24 weeks and was asked about global efficacy at 12 and 24 weeks.

Follow-up: 24 weeks

Endpoints: Primary outcome: mean score for questions related to frequency of penetration and maintenance of an erection after penetration from the IIEF[2] at 0, 12, and 24 weeks (on a 5-point Likert scale, with higher scores reflecting better erectile function). Secondary outcomes: global efficacy as a yes-or-no response to the question "Did the treatment improve your erections?"; adverse events.

RESULTS:

- 465 of 532 (87%) men randomized (285 of 316 in the three sildenafil groups and 180 of 216 in the placebo group) were included in the final analyses.
- Patient characteristics across groups were comparable, with mean ages of approximately 58 years, a 3-year or greater duration of ED, and mainly organic etiology of ED (78%).
- Higher doses of sildenafil resulted in higher mean score for frequency of penetration and maintenance of erection (Table 43.1).
- The rates of treatment discontinuation for any cause (including insufficient response) was 17% in the placebo group, compared to 15%, 7%, and 7% in the 25-mg, 50-mg, and 100-mg groups, respectively.

- The rate of treatment discontinuation due to treatment-related adverse events was 2% in the sildenafil 100-mg arm and 1% in the 25-mg and 50-mg groups.
- The most common side effects were headaches (18%), flushing (18%), dyspepsia (6%), rhinitis (5%), and visual disturbances (2%). Rates of adverse events were strongly correlated to the dose taken.

Table 43.1 SUMMARY OF THE TRIAL'S KEY FINDINGS

	Baseline	Final Score (24 weeks)
Frequency of penetration (per question on IIEF scale)		
Placebo	2.1 ± 0.1	2.2 ± 0.2
25 mg	2.0 ± 0.2	3.2 ± 0.2
50 mg	1.9 ± 0.2	3.5 ± 0.2
100 mg	2.0 ± 0.2	4.0 ± 0.2
Maintenance of erection after penetration (per question on IIEF scale)		
Placebo	1.7 ± 0.1	2.1 ± 0.2
25 mg	1.4 ± 0.1	3.1 ± 0.2
50 mg	1.5 ± 0.1	3.5 ± 0.2
100 mg	1.7 ± 0.1	3.9 ± 0.2

Criticism and Limitations: Participants were instructed not to consume more than two alcoholic drinks within 1 hour of sexual activity, which may limit the generalizability of study findings. The trial's sample size was too small and the follow-up was too short to fully assess the safety profile of sildenafil.

Other Relevant Studies and Information:

- The same publication reported results of a second, two-armed dose-escalation trial in which patients were initially randomized to 50 mg sildenafil or placebo and had the opportunity to increase or reduce the dose based on the perceived response. At the end of the trial, 74% of men in the sildenafil group were taking the highest dose of 100 mg and 10% discontinued medication use for a variety of reasons, including adverse events and lack of efficacy.[1]
- A subsequent trial has found sildenafil to be similarly effective in men with ED due to diabetes.[3]
- Subsequent studies have found sildenafil to be largely safe.[4] Men at particular risk are those with coronary artery disease taking nitrates for angina; this is now recognized as a an absolute contraindication for its use.

- Vardenafil[5] and tadalafil[6] are two other phosphodiesterase-5 (PDE-5) inhibitors used to treat ED. Sildenafil and vardenafil have a very similar absorption time of about 1 hour, a similar half-life of 4 hours, and similar side-effect profiles. Tadalafil has a slower absorption of 2-plus hours but has a half-life of 18 hours.
- The role of PDE-5 inhibitors for penile rehabilitation after radical prostatectomy remains unproven.[7]

Summary and Implications: This study established sildenafil as an effective, reasonably well-tolerated treatment for men with ED of varying etiologies. Overall, the results of the efficacy assessments demonstrate that sildenafil substantially improves erectile function and success rates of intercourse, with effectiveness maintained for at least 6 months. Although adverse effects such as headache, facial flushing, dyspepsia, and visual disturbances were relatively frequent, they are usually transient in nature.

CLINICAL CASE: SILDENAFIL FOR ED

Case History:

A 62-year-old man with past medical history of cigarette smoking and hypertension presents with a 2-year history of gradually worsening erectile function. He has trouble both attaining and maintaining erections. The results of hormonal studies, including testosterone and prolactin, are normal. What options should be offered to him for treatment of his ED?

Suggested Answer:

Based on current guidelines, an oral PDE-5 inhibitor should be first-line treatment for this patient.[8,9] Men in this situation are very likely to respond favorably to sildenafil with improved sexual function. All available PDE-5 inhibitors appear to have similarly efficacy and tolerability, with tadalafil being effective longer, which may help with sexual spontaneity. It is recognized that ED is frequently a symptom of a systemic problem, so attention should be paid to identifying and correcting any modifiable risk factors such as smoking, diabetes, hypertension, obesity, sedentary lifestyle, and hyperlipidemia. Men with three or more of these risk factors may be considered at increased risk for myocardial infarction during sexual activity.[10]

References

1. Goldstein I, Lue TF, Padma-Nathan H, et al. Oral sildenafil in the treatment of erectile dysfunction. Sildenafil Study Group. *N Engl J Med* 1998;338(20):1397–404. doi: 10.1056/NEJM199805143382001

2. Rosen RC, Riley A, Wagner G, Osterloh IH, Kirkpatrick J, Mishra A. The international index of erectile function (IIEF): a multidimensional scale for assessment of erectile dysfunction. *Urology*. 1997;49(6):822–30.

3. Rendell MS, Rajfer J, Wicker PA, et al. Sildenafil for treatment of erectile dysfunction in men with diabetes: a randomized controlled trial. Sildenafil Diabetes Study Group. *JAMA* 1999;281(5):421–6. doi: 10.1001/jama.281.5.421 [published online first: 1999/02/10]

4. Zusman RM, Morales A, Glasser DB, et al. Overall cardiovascular profile of sildenafil citrate. *Am J Cardiol* 1999;83(5A):35C–44C. doi: 10.1016/s0002-9149(99)00046-6 [published online first: 1999/03/17]

5. Hellstrom WJ, Bennett AH, Gesundheit N, et al. A double-blind, placebo-controlled evaluation of the erectile response to transurethral alprostadil. *Urology* 1996;48(6):851–6. doi: 10.1016/s0090-4295(96)00428-1 [published online first: 1996/12/01]

6. Brock GB, McMahon CG, Chen KK, et al. Efficacy and safety of tadalafil for the treatment of erectile dysfunction: results of integrated analyses. *J Urol* 2002;168(4 Pt 1):1332–6. doi: 10.1097/01.ju.0000028041.27703.da [published online first: 2002/09/28]

7. Philippou YA, Jung JH, Steggall MJ, et al. Penile rehabilitation for postprostatectomy erectile dysfunction. *Cochrane Database Syst Rev* 2018;10:CD012414. doi: 10.1002/14651858.CD012414.pub2 [published online first: 2018/10/24]

8. Burnett AL, Nehra A, Breau RH, et al. Erectile dysfunction: AUA guideline. *J Urol* 2018;200(3):633–41. doi: 10.1016/j.juro.2018.05.004 [published online first: 2018/05/11]

9. Hatzimouratidis K, Amar E, Eardley I, et al. Guidelines on male sexual dysfunction: erectile dysfunction and premature ejaculation. *Eur Urol* 2010;57(5):804–14. doi: 10.1016/j.eururo.2010.02.020 [published online first: 2010/03/02]

10. National Cholesterol Education Program Expert Panel on Detection, Evaluation, and Treatment of High Blood Cholesterol in Adults. Adult Treatment Panel III final report. *Circulation* 2002;106(25):3143–421. [published online first: 2002/12/18]

44

Treatment of Men With Erectile Dysfunction With Transurethral Alprostadil

JOSHUA BODIE

"In men with erectile dysfunction, transurethral alprostadil therapy resulted in erections in the clinic and in intercourse at home."[1]

Research Question: In men with chronic erectile dysfunction (ED), how does transurethral alprostadil compare to placebo in achieving erections sufficient for intercourse?

Funding: Supported in part by a grant from Vivus, Inc.

Year Study Began: 1996

Year Study Published: 1997

Study Location: 58 investigational sites in the United States

Who Was Studied: Men in a stable, monogamous, heterosexual relationship unable to achieve a spontaneous erection sufficient for intercourse at any time within the preceding 3 months. All men were considered to have ED of a primarily organic cause based on history, exam, and additional studies such as penile Doppler ultrasound.

Who Was Excluded: Men with a history of urethral stricture or obstruction; those who had a urethral catheter, penile implant, or prior penile surgery; those who had hypogonadism or medical conditions such as diabetes

Patients: 1,511

Study Overview:

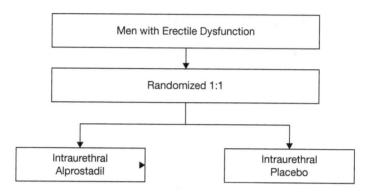

Study Interventions: The study used an active drug run-in period with at least two visits with blinding of both the patients and study personnel. Men were randomized to either a 125-µg or a 250-µg dose at the first visit and then received the other dose level at the next study visit. Initial non-responders underwent the same dose-finding study using dosages of 500 µg and 1,000 µg. Men who did not respond to these higher doses were excluded from the study. In the main trial phase, patients in the intervention arm were given the lowest dose level that had provided a maximal penile response. Alprostadil was administered to the distal urethra by a proprietary drug-delivery system (Medicated Urethral System for Erection [MUSE]) that applied a semisolid pellet of medication. In the control arm a placebo pellet was delivered.

Follow-up: 3 months

Endpoints: There was no prespecified primary endpoint. Participant and partner documentation of response on a scale of 1 to 5 (1 denoted no response; 2, some enlargement; 3, full enlargement (but insufficient rigidity); 4, erection sufficient for intercourse; and 5, full rigidity), the occurrence of sexual intercourse (vaginal penetration), whether the man reached orgasm, the overall level of comfort associated with the use of the medication, and adverse effects noted by the participant or his partner.

RESULTS:

- 515 men did not respond to any dose level in the run-in period in clinic and were excluded upfront.
- The mean patient age was 61 years (range 27 to 88) and the mean partners' age was 56 (range 22 to 84); the mean duration of ED was approximately 4 years and 61.1% reported partial erection at baseline.
- Sexual intercourse was reported as having occurred at least once by 299 (64.9%) of the 461 men in the alprostadil group versus 93 (18.6%) of the 500 men in the placebo group (p < 0.001).
- 293 (63.6%) of the 461 men in the alprostadil group versus 118 (23.6%) of the 500 men in the placebo group experienced orgasm (p < 0.001).
- Intraurethral alprostadil was effective across subgroups based on presumed etiology of ED and patient age.
- Penile pain was reported by 35.7% of men during clinic testing; 2.4% of men discontinued the trial for that reason.
- Dizziness (but no syncope events) was reported by 1.9% of men in the alprostadil group; there were no priapism events.

Criticism and Limitations: This study used an active run-in period that resulted in over one-third of participants being excluded upfront. Give the high incidence of drug-related penile pain, it is doubtful whether patient blinding was successfully maintained.

Other Relevant Studies and Information:

- An analysis based on the Massachusetts Male Aging Study in men 40 to 70 years of age found a combined prevalence of minimal, moderate, and complete impotence of 52%. The prevalence of complete impotence tripled from 5% to 15% between subject ages 40 and 70 years.[2]
- Subsequent trials have confirmed similar effectiveness of intraurethral alprostadil.[3–5]
- Trials have demonstrated the effectiveness of intracavernosal alprostadil injections,[6] which may be preferred by patients over intraurethral application.[7]
- Major guidelines recommend intraurethral alprostadil as an alternative to phosphodiesterase-5 (PDE-5) inhibitors, vacuum erection devices, and intracavernosal injections.[8,9]

Summary and Implications: At the time the study was published, the treatment options for ED included oral supplements with limited efficacy (such as yohimbine), vacuum erection devices, penile prosthesis surgery, vascular surgery, and intracavernosal injections. This study describes the initial experience with transurethral alprostadil and identified the effectiveness of patient-specific doses. The use of locally applied drugs, without needles, continues to be an appealing way to treat ED.

CLINICAL CASE: INTRAURETHRAL ALPROSTADIL FOR ED

Case History:

Four months after undergoing bilateral nerve-sparing robotic-assisted laparoscopic prostatectomy (RALP), a patient presents with persistent ED refractory to oral PDE-5 inhibitors. He has achieved excellent continence results, and he and his partner are keen to resume sexual relations. What can you offer him?

Suggested Answer:

This patient can hope to experience further improvement of his erectile function at least up to 1 year after undergoing RALP. Given that he has not responded to PDE-5 inhibitors as first-line therapy, intraurethral alprostadil is an alternative to intracavernosal injections in patients who prefer a less-invasive therapy.[8,9] It is recommended that these patients undergo an in-office test to teach them the appropriate application technique and for dose-finding purposes. They should be educated about the risk of priapism, although the risk with intraurethral application of alprostadil appears to be low. Common adverse events are genital pain (up to 35%), urethral pain or burning (up to 29%), and dizziness (up to 7.0%). Penile prosthesis implantation is typically reserved for men who have failed or are unwilling to consider less invasive alternatives.

References

1. Padma-Nathan H, Hellstrom WJ, Kaiser FE, et al. Treatment of men with erectile dysfunction with transurethral alprostadil. Medicated Urethral System for Erection (MUSE) Study Group. *N Engl J Med* 1997;336(1):1–7. doi: 10.1056/NEJM199701023360101
2. Feldman HA, Goldstein I, Hatzichristou DG, et al. Impotence and its medical and psychosocial correlates: results of the Massachusetts Male Aging Study. *J Urol*

1994;151(1):54–61. doi: 10.1016/s0022-5347(17)34871-1 [published online first: 1994/01/01]

3. Williams G, Abbou CC, Amar ET, et al. The effect of transurethral alprostadil on the quality of life of men with erectile dysfunction, and their partners. MUSE Study Group. *Br J Urol* 1998;82(6):847–54. doi: 10.1046/j.1464-410x.1998.00937.x [published online first: 1999/01/12]

4. Hellstrom WJ, Bennett AH, Gesundheit N, et al. A double-blind, placebo-controlled evaluation of the erectile response to transurethral alprostadil. *Urology* 1996;48(6):851–6. doi: 10.1016/s0090-4295(96)00428-1 [published online first: 1996/12/01]

5. Peterson CA, Bennett AH, Hellstrom WJ, et al. Erectile response to trans-urethral alprostadil, prazosin and alprostadil-prazosin combinations. *J Urol* 1998;159(5):1523–7; discussion 27–8. doi: 10.1097/00005392-199805000-00030 [published online first: 1998/04/29]

6. Linet OI, Ogrinc FG. Efficacy and safety of intracavernosal alprostadil in men with erectile dysfunction. The Alprostadil Study Group. *N Engl J Med* 1996;334(14):873–7. doi: 10.1056/NEJM199604043341401 [published online first: 1996/04/04]

7. Shabsigh R, Padma-Nathan H, Gittleman M, et al. Intracavernous alprostadil alfadex is more efficacious, better tolerated, and preferred over intraurethral alprostadil plus optional ACTIS: a comparative, randomized, crossover, multicenter study. *Urology* 2000;55(1):109–13. doi: 10.1016/s0090-4295(99)00442-2 [published online first: 2000/02/02]

8. Burnett AL, Nehra A, Breau RH, et al. Erectile dysfunction: AUA guideline. *J Urol* 2018;200(3):633–41. doi: 10.1016/j.juro.2018.05.004 [published online first: 2018/05/11]

9. Hatzimouratidis K, Amar E, Eardley I, et al. Guidelines on male sexual dysfunction: erectile dysfunction and premature ejaculation. *Eur Urol* 2010;57(5):804–14. doi: 10.1016/j.eururo.2010.02.020 [published online first: 2010/03/02]

45

Antimicrobial Prophylaxis for Children With Vesicoureteral Reflux

Randomized Intervention for Children With Vesicoureteral Reflux (RIVUR) Trial

PHILIPP DAHM AND JANE M. LEWIS

> "Among children with vesicoureteral reflux after urinary tract infection, antimicrobial prophylaxis was associated with a substantially reduced risk of recurrence but not of renal scarring."[1]

Research Question: In children with vesicoureteral reflux (VUR) diagnosed after a first or second febrile or symptomatic urinary tract infection (UTI), is trimethoprim–sulfamethoxazole (TMP-SMX) prophylaxis effective in preventing recurrences?

Funding: Funded by the National Institute of Diabetes and Digestive and Kidney Diseases (and others)

Year Study Began: June 2007

Year Study Published: June 2014

Study Location: Nineteen pediatric tertiary care centers in the United States

Who Was Studied: Children under the age of 6 years with grade I to IV VUR and one or two febrile or symptomatic UTIs within 112 days prior to randomization

Who Was Excluded: Children with grade V reflux, no prior febrile or symptomatic UTIs, and those with coexisting urological anomalies

Patients: 607

Study Overview:

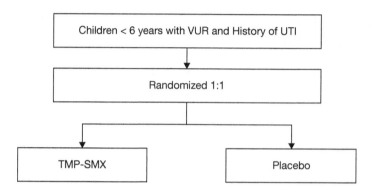

Study Interventions: Children in the intervention arm received daily TMP-SMX suspension (3 mg/kg TMP plus 15 mg/kg SMX). Children in the control arm received placebo that was nearly identical in color, smell, taste, and consistency. Urine specimens from children who were not toilet trained were obtained by catheterization or suprapubic aspiration; bag-collected specimens were not permitted. Clean, voided specimens were collected from toilet-trained children. Index and outcome infections were defined as evidence of pyuria on urinalysis, culture-proven infection, and fever (at least 38°C) or urinary tract symptoms within 24 hours before or after urine collection. Renal scanning with technetium-99m–labeled dimercaptosuccinic acid (DMSA) was performed at baseline and after 1 and 2 years to assess for renal scarring.

Follow-up: 24 months

Endpoints: Primary outcome: febrile or symptomatic UTI recurrence. Secondary outcomes: renal scarring, failure of prophylaxis, and antimicrobial resistance. The trial also assessed bladder and bowel dysfunction using standardized measures.

RESULTS:

- The mean patient age was 12 months and 91.9% were girls; 484 (80.4%) of the 602 children had grade II or III reflux.
- The vast majority of patients (91.3%) had experienced one prior UTI; in 53.5% this was described as febrile and symptomatic.
- TMP prophylaxis reduced the rate of recurrent febrile or symptomatic UTI by 11.9% (95% confidence interval [CI], 4.6 to 19.2) but did not reduce renal scarring (Table 45.1).
- Antimicrobial resistance was substantially more common in the antibiotic prophylaxis group.

Table 45.1 SUMMARY OF THE RIVUR TRIAL FINDINGS

Outcome	TMP-SMX	Placebo	Absolute Risk Reduction (95% CI)
Recurrent febrile or symptomatic UTI	25.5%	37.4%	11.9% (4.6 to 19.2)
Renal scarring (overall)	11.9%	10.2%	−1.7% (−7.4 to 4.0)
Recurrent febrile or symptomatic UTI by any resistant pathogen	68.4%	24.6%	−43.8% (−61.7 to −25.8)

Criticism and Limitations: The study enrolled children with a prior UTI rather than children with incidentally detected cases of VUR. It used a composite primary outcome of febrile and symptomatic UTI. Subsequent studies have questioned this practice.[2]

Other Relevant Studies and Information:

- Another methodologically rigorous and similar study from Australia, the Prevention of Recurrent Urinary Tract Infection in Children with Vesicoureteric Reflux and Normal Renal Tracts (PRIVENT) trial, found a 6% absolute risk reduction in favor of antibiotic prophylaxis in reducing UTIs.[3]
- Correspondingly, major urological guidelines recommend antibiotic prophylaxis in children less than 1 year of age with VUR and a history of a febrile UTI.[4,5] They also recommend antibiotic prophylaxis in screen-detected cases of VUR grade III to V.

- In contrast, a recent Cochrane review concluded that low-dose antibiotic prophylaxis compared to no treatment/placebo may make little or no difference to the risk of repeat symptomatic UTI (risk ratio [RR] 0.77, 95% CI, 0.54 to 1.09; low certainty evidence) and febrile UTI (RR 0.83, 95% CI, 0.56 to 1.21; low certainty evidence) at 1 to 2 years.[2]
- A meta-analysis of six trials limited to febrile infants aged 2 to 24 months also did not find antibiotic prophylaxis to be effective. Citing this study, the American Academy of Pediatrics recommends prompt treatment of a UTI rather than continued prophylaxis.[6]

Summary and Implications: Together with the PRIVENT study[3] as the two most methodologically rigorous trials, this study provides the underpinning for the guideline of the American Urological Association that advocates for low-dose antibiotic prophylaxis for the first year of life. As reflected by contradictory urological[4,5] and pediatric guidelines,[6] however, this remains an area of considerable controversy.

CLINICAL CASE: LONG-TERM ANTIBIOTIC PROPHYLAXIS IN CHILDREN WITH VUR

Case History:

A 6-month-old female is brought to the pediatrician by her parents, who report unusual irritability, refusal to eat, and crying when wetting into her diaper. A urinalysis obtained by catherization demonstrates bacteria, leukocytes, and positive leukocyte esterase and nitrite. The child is treated empirically with a 7-day course of antibiotics; a urine culture later confirms an *Escherichia coli* infection. A renal ultrasound reveals left-sided, moderate hydronephrosis. A subsequent voiding cystourethrogram indicates right-sided grade I VUR and left-sided grade III VUR.

Suggested Answer:

Based on current American Urological Association guidelines,[4] the parents would be recommended to start prophylaxis with either nitrofurantoin or SMX-TMP and continue until the child is 12 months old. At this point, repeat renal ultrasound would be performed to assess for appropriate renal growth. If kidney sizes are asymmetric, prophylaxis should be continued and a DMSA renal scan should be considered to evaluate propensity for renal scarring. If kidneys are symmetric in size, the clinician should discuss with the parents the pros and cons of ongoing prophylaxis and arrive at a shared decision about continued use or discontinuation.

References

1. RIVUR Trial Investigators. Antimicrobial prophylaxis for children with vesicoureteral reflux. *N Engl J Med* 2014;370(25):2367–76. doi: 10.1056/NEJMoa1401811

2. Williams G, Hodson EM, Craig JC. Interventions for primary vesicoureteric reflux. *Cochrane Database Syst Rev* 2019;2:CD001532. doi: 10.1002/14651858.CD001532. pub5 [published online first: 2019/02/21]

3. Craig JC, Simpson JM, Williams GJ, et al. Antibiotic prophylaxis and recurrent urinary tract infection in children. *N Engl J Med* 2009;361(18):1748–59. doi: 10.1056/NEJMoa0902295 [published online first: 2009/10/30]

4. Peters CA, Skoog SJ, Arant BS, Jr., et al. Summary of the AUA guideline on management of primary vesicoureteral reflux in children. *J Urol* 2010;184(3):1134–44. doi: 10.1016/j.juro.2010.05.065 [published online first: 2010/07/24]

5. Tekgul S, Riedmiller H, Hoebeke P, et al. EAU guidelines on vesicoureteral reflux in children. *Eur Urol* 2012;62(3):534–42. doi: 10.1016/j.eururo.2012.05.059 [published online first: 2012/06/16]

6. American Academy of Pediatrics. Reaffirmation of AAP clinical practice guideline: The diagnosis and management of the initial urinary tract infection in febrile infants and young children 2–24 months of age. *Pediatrics* 2016;138(6):e20163026.

46

A Comparison of Transurethral Surgery With Watchful Waiting for Moderate Symptoms of Benign Prostatic Hyperplasia

The Veterans Affairs Cooperative Study Group on Transurethral Resection of the Prostate

JAE HUNG JUNG

"For men with moderate symptoms of benign prostatic hyperplasia, surgery is more effective than watchful waiting in reducing the rate of treatment failure and improving genitourinary symptoms."[1]

Research Question: In men with moderate symptoms of benign prostatic hyperplasia (BPH), how do transurethral resection of prostate (TURP) and watchful waiting (WW) compare?

Funding: Supported by the Cooperative Studies Program of the Department of Veterans Affairs Medical Research Service

Year Study Began: 1986

Year Study Published: 1995

Study Location: 11 Veterans Affairs Medical Centers in the United States

Who Was Studied: Male veterans over the age of 55 years with moderate to severe lower urinary tract symptoms (LUTS), which were assessed using a scale from 0 to 27 (with higher scores indicating worse symptoms) based on a nine-question interview. Patients with a score between 10 to 20 were eligible for enrollment.

Who Was Excluded: Men under the age of 55; those with a prior history of prostate surgery or pelvic radiation treatment, a postvoid residual of more than 350 cc, or a serum creatinine concentration higher than 3.0 mg/dl; and those with serious medical conditions making them unfit for surgery

Patients: 556

Study Overview:

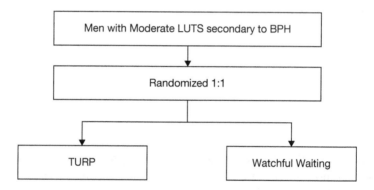

Study Interventions: Patients in the intervention arm underwent TURP performed by a staff surgeon or the chief surgical resident within 2 weeks after randomization. Patients in the control arm (WW) were advised to avoid ingesting coffee, alcohol, and other liquids after dinner and were informed about medications that might make their symptoms worse. Physicians were asked to avoid prescribing medications such as alpha-adrenergic antagonists that might confound the results of the trial.

Follow-up: Average follow-up was 2.8 years.

Endpoints: Primary outcome: treatment failure, defined as the occurrence of death, retention, bladder stone, doubling of baseline serum creatine, new-onset incontinence, or American Urological Association symptom score (International Prostate Symptom Score [IPSS]) of 24 or higher at one visit (or scores of 21 or higher at two consecutive visits)

RESULTS:

- The mean patient age was approximately 66 years and the mean symptom score at study entry was 14.6.
- 249 (89%) of the 280 men randomized to the intervention arm underwent TURP. The median weight of prostatic tissue removed was 14 g (25th percentile, 8 g; 75th percentile, 21 g). Seventy-eight percent of the patients were hospitalized for 4 days or less after surgery (4 ± 4 days).
- There were 23 treatment failures in the TURP group compared with 47 in the WW group (relative risk [RR], 0.48; 95% confidence interval [CI], 0.30 to 0.77) (Table 46.1).
- Of the 276 men assigned to the WW group, 65 (24%) underwent surgery within 3 years after the assignment.
- 9% of the men in the TURP group experienced a perioperative complication; the most common complications were need for catheter replacement (4%), prostate capsule perforation (2%), and bleeding requiring transfusion (1%).
- Mortality rates over 3 years were similar at 1.7% and 1.3% in the TURP and WW group, respectively.
- TURP was associated with improved symptoms and improved scores for bother from urinary difficulties and interference with the activities of daily living, improved peak flow rate, and a decreased volume of residual urine.

Table 46.1 EVENTS THAT CONTRIBUTED TO TREATMENT FAILURE

Outcome	Surgery (n = 280)	Watchful Waiting (n = 276)	Relative Risk (95% CI)
Treatment failure	23 (8.2%)	47 (17.2%)	0.48 (0.30 – 0.77)
Death	13 (4.6%)	10 (3.6%)	1.28 (0.57 – 2.87)
Urinary retention	1 (0.3%)	8 (2.9%)	0.12 (0.02 – 0.98)
High residual urinary volume	3 (1.1%)	16 (5.8%)	0.18 (0.05 – 0.63)
Renal azotemia	3 (1.1%)	1 (0.4%)	2.96 (0.31 – 28.26)
Bladder stones	0 (0%)	1 (0.4%)	0.00
Persistent incontinence	4 (1.4%)	4 (1.5%)	0.99 (0.25 – 3.90)
High symptom score	1 (0.3%)	12 (4.3%)	0.08 (0.01 – 0.63)
Prostate adenocarcinoma	24 (8.6%)	8 (2.9%)	2.96 (1.35 – 6.47)

Criticism and Limitations: The study made no attempt to blind patients, study personnel, or outcome assessors. The primary outcome was a composite outcome that included components of very different importance to patients (spanning from death to high postvoid residuals).[2] The crossover from the WW to the TURP group was high (24%). Surgical technique and perioperative care (including length of stay) differed considerably from today's standard of care, thereby limiting applicability to modern practice. TURP was compared to WW rather than medical therapy with agents commonly used as first-line therapy today, in particular alpha-blockers.

Other Relevant Studies and Information:

- In a 5-year follow-up study, treatment failure rates were 10% for TURP versus 21% for WW (RR 0.476, 95% CI, 0.313 to 0.724).[3] The crossover rate to TURP in the WW group at 5 years was 36% and was positively associated with the degree of bother.
- A cost-effectiveness analysis from 1988 using a base case of a 70-year-old man with moderate symptom severity found immediate TURP to be associated with a 1.0-month loss of life expectancy and a gain in 2.9 quality-adjusted life months, emphasizing the importance of patient preferences in decision making.[4]
- Alpha-blockers, 5-alpha-reductase inhibitors, and phosphodiesterase inhibitors have all since been added to the conservative treatment armamentarium for male LUTS due to BPH.[5]
- Whereas TURP remains the "gold standard" for the surgical treatment of male LUTS, a large number of alternative treatment modalities have since become available[6] and are listed as options in the American Urological Association guidelines.[5] These include various laser ablation and enucleation procedures, Aquablation,[7] the prostatic urethral lift procedure,[8] and convective water vapor energy therapy.[9]

Summary and Implications: This study helped to establish TURP as the "gold standard" surgical treatment for men with LUTS.

CLINICAL CASE: TURP IN MEN WITH LUTS ATTRIBUTED TO BPH

Case History:

A 66-year-old male presents with a 2-year history of worsening LUTS that include a weak stream, postvoid dribbling, frequency, and nocturia two times a night. His IPSS is 18 and he reports a quality-of-life score of "terrible." He has stopped drinking caffeinated beverages and reduced his evening fluid intake.

He was prescribed tamsulosin by his primary care doctor but had to stop it because of lightheadedness. His past medical history is only notable for hypertension. His prostate size is approximately 40 g per digital rectal exam, his maximum urinary flow is 7.6 ml/sec, and his postvoid residual is repeatedly around 100 ml. Should he be offered a TURP?

Suggested Answer:

This patient has failed behavioral modification and was unable to tolerate an alpha-blocker. Given his prostate size of less than 50 g, he is unlikely to gain much benefit from treatment with a 5-alpha-reductase inhibitor, which would take a prolonged time to take effect. He is likely to experience substantial improvement in terms of symptom score, quality of life, flow rate, and postvoid residuals by undergoing a TURP. Whereas a number of alternative procedures with different effect profiles have become available (e.g., Aquablation, prostatic urethral lift, and convective water vapor energy ablation), these are much less established. A TURP continues to be a guideline-concordant treatment choice.[5,10,11]

References

1. Wasson JH, Reda DJ, Bruskewitz RC, et al. A comparison of transurethral surgery with watchful waiting for moderate symptoms of benign prostatic hyperplasia. The Veterans Affairs Cooperative Study Group on Transurethral Resection of the Prostate. N Engl J Med 1995;332(2):75–9. doi: 10.1056/NEJM199501123320202

2. Montori VM, Permanyer-Miralda G, Ferreira-Gonzalez I, et al. Validity of composite end points in clinical trials. BMJ 2005;330(7491):594–6.

3. Flanigan RC, Reda DJ, Wasson JH, et al. 5-year outcome of surgical resection and watchful waiting for men with moderately symptomatic benign prostatic hyperplasia: a Department of Veterans Affairs cooperative study. J Urol 1998;160(1):12–6; discussion 16–7. [published online first: 1998/06/17]

4. Barry MJ, Mulley AG, Jr., Fowler FJ, et al. Watchful waiting vs immediate transurethral resection for symptomatic prostatism. The importance of patients' preferences. JAMA 1988;259(20):3010–7. [published online first: 1988/05/27]

5. Foster HE, Dahm P, Kohler TS, et al. Surgical management of lower urinary tract symptoms attributed to benign prostatic hyperplasia: AUA guideline amendment 2019. J Urol 2019;202(3):592–8. doi: 10.1097/JU.0000000000000319 [published online first: 2019/05/07]

6. Dahm P, Jung JH. The promise of new urological procedures and medications to manage lower urinary tract symptoms related to benign prostatic obstruction. Curr Opin Urol 2018;28(3):260–1. doi: 10.1097/MOU.0000000000000493 [published online first: 2018/03/15]

7. Hwang EC, Jung JH, Borofsky M, et al. Aquablation of the prostate for the treatment of lower urinary tract symptoms in men with benign prostatic hyperplasia. Cochrane

Database Syst Rev 2019;2:CD013143. doi: 10.1002/14651858.CD013143.pub2 [published online first: 2019/02/14]

8. Jung JH, Reddy B, McCutcheon KA, et al. Prostatic urethral lift for the treatment of lower urinary tract symptoms in men with benign prostatic hyperplasia. *Cochrane Database Syst Rev* 2019;5:CD012832. doi: 10.1002/14651858.CD012832.pub2 [published online first: 2019/05/28]

9. Kang TW, Jung JH, Hwang EC, et al. Convective radiofrequency water vapour thermal therapy for lower urinary tract symptoms in men with benign prostatic hyperplasia. *Cochrane Database Syst Rev* 2020;3:CD013251. doi: 10.1002/14651858. CD013251.pub2 [published online first: 2020/03/27]

10. Nickel JC, Aaron L, Barkin J, et al. Canadian Urological Association guideline on male lower urinary tract symptoms/benign prostatic hyperplasia (MLUTS/BPH): 2018 update. *Can Urol Assoc J* 2018;12(10):303–12. doi: 10.5489/cuaj.5616 [published online first: 2018/10/18]

11. Oelke M, Bachmann A, Descazeaud A, et al. EAU guidelines on the treatment and follow-up of non-neurogenic male lower urinary tract symptoms including benign prostatic obstruction. *Eur Urol* 2013;64(1):118–40. doi: 10.1016/ j.eururo.2013.03.004 [published online first: 2013/04/02]

47

The Efficacy of Terazosin, Finasteride, or Both in Benign Prostatic Hyperplasia

The Veterans Affairs Cooperative Benign Prostatic Hyperplasia Study

JAE HUNG JUNG

"In men with benign prostatic hyperplasia, terazosin was effective therapy, whereas finasteride was not, and the combination of terazosin and finasteride was no more effective than terazosin alone."[1]

Research Question: In patients with lower urinary tract symptoms (LUTS) attributed to benign prostatic hyperplasia (BPH), how do terazosin, finasteride, and their combination compare?

Funding: The Cooperative Studies Program of the Department of Veterans Affairs Medical Research Service, Merck and Co., and Abbott Laboratories

Year Study Began: 1992

Year Study Published: 1996

Study Location: Multiple Veterans Affairs Medical Centers in the United States

Who Was Studied: Men 45 to 80 years of age with an American Urological Association symptom score (AUA-SS) of at least 8, a mean peak urinary flow rate (Q_{max}) of no more than 15 ml/sec and no less than 4 ml/sec, a minimal voided volume of 125 ml, and a mean residual volume after voiding of less than 300 ml

Who Was Excluded: Patients who had taken terazosin, finasteride, or an anticholinergic or any antihypertensive drug except a diuretic or an angiotensin-converting enzyme inhibitor within 2 weeks before the lead-in period; patients who had taken an estrogen, androgen, or drug causing androgen inhibition within the preceding 3 months

Patients: 1,229

Study Overview:

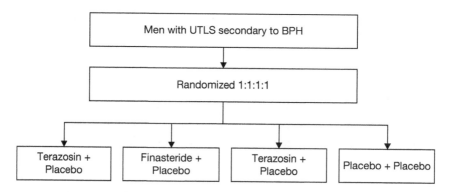

Study Interventions: Participants received one of four regimens. The terazosin group received terazosin (titration schedule: days 1 to 3, 1 mg; days 4 to 7, 2 mg; days 8 to 14, 5 mg; and day 15 through the completion of the study, 10 mg) and finasteride placebo single daily at bedtime. The finasteride group received 5 mg finasteride and terazosin placebo single daily at bedtime. The combination therapy group received terazosin and finasteride single daily at bedtime. The placebo group received terazosin and finasteride placebos single daily at bedtime.

Follow-up: 52 weeks

Endpoints: Primary outcomes: AUA-SS and Q_{max}. Secondary outcomes: compliance and adverse events.

RESULTS:

- Mean changes in the AUA-SS at 52 weeks were decreases of 2.6 points in the placebo group, 3.2 points in the finasteride group, 6.1 points in the terazosin group, and 6.2 points in the combination therapy group.
- Mean changes in Q_{max} at 52 weeks in the placebo, finasteride, terazosin, and combination therapy groups were increases of 1.4, 1.6, 2.7, and 3.2 ml/sec, respectively.
- Comparing finasteride alone, terazosin alone, and combination therapy to placebo, results (calculated from reported data) are shown in Table 47.1.
- Reported adverse events are summarized in Table 47.2. Dizziness and impotence were the most commonly reported adverse events for terazosin and finasteride, respectively.

Table 47.1 KEY STUDY FINDINGS COMPARING FINASTERIDE, TERAZOSIN, AND THEIR COMBINATION TO PLACEBO

	Finasteride MD (95% CI)	Rate ratio (95% CI)	Terazosin MD (95% CI)	Rate ratio (95% CI)	Combination MD (95% CI)	Rate ratio (95% CI)
AUA-SS	−0.20 (−0.25 to −0.15)	–	−3.00 (−3.05 to −2.95)	–	−3.40 (−3.45 to −3.35)	–
Q_{max} (ml/sec)	0.30 (0.25 to 0.35)	–	1.40 (1.35 to 1.45)	–	1.80 (1.75 to 1.85)	–
Prostatic volume (cm³)	−8.80 (−8.92 to −8.68)	–	−0.90 (−1.01 to −0.79)	–	−8.70 (−8.81 to −8.59)	–
Adverse events	–	1.45 (1.40 to 1.50)	–	2.27 (2.20 to 2.34)	–	2.64 (2.57 to 2.72)

95% CI, 95% confidence interval.

Table 47.2 MOST COMMON ADVERSE EVENTS COMPARING FINASTERIDE, TERAZOSIN, AND THEIR COMBINATION TO PLACEBO

Outcome	Placebo (n = 305)	Finasteride (n = 310)	Terazosin (n = 305)	Combination (n = 309)
Dizziness	22	26	79	66
Postural hypotension	3	7	23	27
Impotence	14	29	18	29
Ejaculatory disorder	4	6	1	21

Criticism and Limitations: This study did not include a threshold prostate size as an eligibility criterion, thereby including men of all prostate sizes (mean size 37 ml). This has been suggested as an explanation for the limited response to finasteride treatment.[2]

Other Relevant Studies and Information:

- In a secondary analysis of men with prostatic volume greater than 50 cm³, the authors found a more pronounced treatment effect in men in the placebo, finasteride, terazosin, and combination groups, with AUA-SS reductions of 2.5, 3.6, 6, and 7 from baseline to study end, respectively.[1]
- A similar, larger study by McConnell et al. with the alpha-blocker doxazosin (instead of terazosin), the Medical Therapy of Prostatic Symptoms (MTOPS) study, has suggested a benefit of combination therapy over alpha-blocker or finasteride use alone.[4]
- Since this study was published, the 5-alpha reductase inhibitor (5-ARI) dutasteride has become available. In the Combination of Avodart and Tamsulosin (CombAT) study, comparing tamsulosin, dutasteride, and combination therapy, mean AUA-SS decreased by 3.8, 5.3, and 6.3 points, respectively, compared to baseline.[5]
- Based on current American Urological Association (AUA)[6] and European Association of Urology[7] guidelines, alpha-blockers are the first-line treatment for male LUTS attributed to BPH.

Summary and Implications: This study demonstrated the benefit of alpha-blocker therapy for men with BPH symptoms but did not demonstrate added benefit of combination alpha-blocker and 5-ARI therapy. Subsequent studies have since demonstrated the value of combination therapy in men with a prostate larger than 40 ml, however.

CLINICAL CASE: ALPHA-BLOCKER ALONE VERSUS COMBINATION THERAPY

Case History:

A 63-year-old patient with no significant medical comorbidities complains of LUTS that have slowly worsened over the year. Complaints include a decreased force of stream, postvoid dribbling, and nocturia once a night, which he finds quite bothersome. He has been previously counseled about behavioral changes such as fluid restriction and avoidance of caffeinated beverages late in the day, but this not yielded any substantial improvement. His AUA-SS is 16 and his QOL is 4. On digital rectal examination his prostate is about 30 g in size and his prostate-specific antigen level is 2.3 ng/ml. What do you recommend?

Suggested Answer:

The results of this study and studies of alpha-blockers used to treat male LUTS indicate that patients can expect an improvement of 4 to 6 points on the AUA-SS with an alpha-blocker alone. Quality of life is also improved, as is urinary stream. An alpha-blocker alone is the preferred medication in this man who does not have a particularly enlarged prostate per his digital rectal exam. Combination therapy is therefore not indicated, based on current AUA guidelines on the medical management of male LUTS[6] as well as those of the EAU.[7] Terazosin used in this trial requires dose titration and blood pressure monitoring but is inexpensive and dosed once daily. It appears to be equally effective to tamsulosin, which is often preferred because dose titration is not required. He should be informed that dizziness is the most common side effect of alpha-blockers and that there is a 10% chance of ejaculatory dysfunction with tamsulosin.

References

1. Lepor H, Williford WO, Barry MJ, et al. The impact of medical therapy on bother due to symptoms, quality of life and global outcome, and factors predicting response. Veterans Affairs Cooperative Studies Benign Prostatic Hyperplasia Study Group. *J Urol.* 1998;160(4):1358–1367.

2. Walsh PC. Treatment of benign prostatic hyperplasia. *N Engl J Med.* 1996;335(8):586–587.

3. Barry MJ, Williford WO, Chang Y, et al. Benign prostatic hyperplasia specific health status measures in clinical research: how much change in the American Urological Association symptom index and the benign prostatic hyperplasia impact index is perceptible to patients? *J Urol.* 1995;154(5):1770–1774.

4. McConnell JD, Roehrborn CG, Bautista OM, et al. The long-term effect of doxazosin, finasteride, and combination therapy on the clinical progression of benign prostatic hyperplasia. *N Engl J Med.* 2003;349(25):2387–2398.

5. Montorsi F, Roehrborn C, Garcia-Penit J, et al. The effects of dutasteride or tamsulosin alone and in combination on storage and voiding symptoms in men with lower urinary tract symptoms (LUTS) and benign prostatic hyperplasia (BPH): 4-year data from the Combination of Avodart and Tamsulosin (CombAT) study. *BJU Int.* 2011;107(9):1426–1431.

6. McVary KT, Roehrborn CG, Avins AL, et al. Update on AUA guideline on the management of benign prostatic hyperplasia. *J Urol.* 2011;185(5):1793–1803.

7. Oelke M, Bachmann A, Descazeaud A, et al. EAU guidelines on the treatment and follow-up of non-neurogenic male lower urinary tract symptoms including benign prostatic obstruction. *Eur Urol.* 2013;64(1):118–140.

Chlorhexidine–Alcohol Versus Povidone–Iodine for Surgical-Site Antisepsis

PHILIPP DAHM

"Preoperative cleansing of the patient's skin with chlorhexidine–alcohol is superior to cleansing with povidone–iodine for preventing surgical-site infection after clean-contaminated surgery."[1]

Research Question: In patients undergoing clean-contaminated surgery, how does chlorhexidine–alcohol scrub compare to povidone–iodine scrub and paint in terms of infection rates?

Funding: Funded in part by Cardinal Health

Year Study Began: April 2004

Year Study Published: May 2008

Study Location: 6 university-affiliated hospitals in the United States

Who Was Studied: Patients 18 years of age or older who were undergoing clean-contaminated surgery—that is, colorectal, small intestinal, gastroesophageal, biliary, thoracic, gynecologic, or urologic operations performed under controlled conditions without substantial spillage or unusual contamination

Who Was Excluded: Patients with a history of allergy to chlorhexidine, alcohol, or iodophors; evidence of infection at or adjacent to the operative site

Patients: 897

Study Overview:

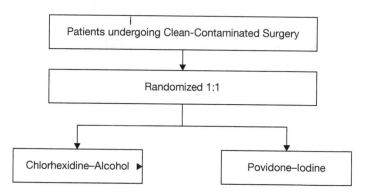

Study Interventions: Patients in the intervention arm had the skin at the surgical site preoperatively scrubbed with an applicator that contained 2% chlorhexidine gluconate and 70% isopropyl alcohol (ChloraPrep, Cardinal Health). Those in the control arm were preoperatively scrubbed and then painted with an aqueous solution of 10% povidone–iodine (Scrub Care Skin Prep Tray, Cardinal Health). More than one chlorhexidine–alcohol applicator was used if the coverage area exceeded 33 × 33 cm. Randomization was stratified by hospital.

Follow-up: 30 days

Endpoints: Primary outcome: any surgical-site infection within 30 days after surgery. Secondary outcomes: individual types of surgical-site infections classified as superficial incisional infection, deep incisional infection, or organ-space infection.

RESULTS:

- The mean patient age was 57 years and all patients received preoperative systemic antibiotics.
- Approximately 70% of patients had abdominal surgery (mostly colorectal but also biliary and small intestinal); approximately 30% underwent

non-abdominal surgery (thoracic, gynecologic, and urologic). The latter contributed approximately 7% of participants.

- Chlorhexidine reduced the rate of any surgical infection (Table 48.1) as well as that of superficial incisional infection, but no difference was observed for deep incisional infection, organ-space infection, and sepsis from surgical-site infection.
- Rates of any type of adverse event (55.7% vs. 58.2%) and serious adverse events (17.6% vs. 15.9%) were similar in the chlorhexidine–alcohol and povidone–iodine groups, respectively.

Table 48.1 PROPORTION OF PATIENTS WITH SURGICAL-SITE INFECTIONS

Type of infection	Chlorhexidine–Alcohol	Povidone–Iodine	Relative Risk (95% CI)
Any surgical site infection	9.5%	16.1%	0.59 (0.41 – 0.85)
Superficial incisional infection	4.2%	8.6%	0.48 (0.28 – 0.84)
Deep incisional infection	1.0%	3.0%	0.33 (0.11 – 1.01)
Organ-space infection	4.4%	4.5%	0.97 (0.52 – 1.80)
Sepsis from surgical-site infection	2.7%	4.3%	0.62 (0.30 – 1.29)

Criticism and Limitations: The study controlled for potential differences in hospital practices that might impact surgical-site infection rates, which was a strength. It was not powered for an analysis of type of infection, and the number of patients undergoing urologic procedures was relatively small. It did not include a comparison arm of chlorhexidine–alcohol.

Other Relevant Studies and Information:

- Another large randomized controlled trial established that chlorhexidine–alcohol was superior to iodine–alcohol in pregnant women undergoing cesarean section in reducing surgical-site infections (hazard ratio 0.55; 95% confidence interval [CI], 0.34 to 0.90).[2]
- A systematic review of five randomized controlled trials found chlorhexidine–alcohol to be superior to aqueous iodophor but found no difference between chlorhexidine–alcohol and iodophor-alcohol.[3]

- A small trial in men with erectile dysfunction undergoing placement of an inflatable penile prothesis found post-preparation skin cultures to be positive in 8% and 32% of participants in the chlorhexidine–alcohol group versus the povidone–iodine group, respectively. No urethral or genital skin complications occurred in either group.[4]
- Guidelines from the Centers for Disease Control and Prevention[5] and the American College of Surgeons[6] recommend intraoperative skin preparation with an antiseptic agent containing alcohol unless contraindicated.

Summary and Implications: This study presents a cornerstone in the body of evidence that supports the superiority of skin preparation using chlorhexidine–alcohol over povidone–iodine, which had previously been the most commonly used form of preoperative skin preparation. It remains uncertain whether other alcohol-based skin preparations are similarly effective.

CLINICAL CASE: CHLORHEXIDINE–ALCOHOL VERSUS POVIDONE–IODINE SKIN PREPARATION IN INFLATABLE PENILE PROSTHESIS (IPP) SURGERY

Case History:

A 70-year-old male undergoes robotic-assisted laparoscopic prostatectomy, which leaves him with persistent erectile dysfunction 18 months later. His erectile dysfunction is not responsive to either phosphodiesterase-5 inhibitors or intraurethral prostaglandin. He is strongly opposed to the idea of intracavernosal injection therapy and chooses placement of an IPP. You explicitly discuss the risk of infection as a potential complication with him. How do you best proceed to minimize the patient's risk?

Suggested Answer:

Measures to reduce perioperative infection risk in patients undergoing IPP include ensuring that the patient has a negative urine culture, removing hair from the operative field, and using an appropriate presurgical hand scrub and perioperative antibiotics.[7] Guidelines by the International Consultation on Sexual Medicine further recommend an alcohol-based skin preparation prior to IPP placement. Based on the trial by Darouiche et al.[1] as well as the trial by Yeung et al.,[4] chlorhexidine–alcohol is the preferred skin preparation in this situation.[8] It is important that the preparation solution is allowed to dry after it is applied and that the IPP is placed using a "no-touch" technique.

References

1. Darouiche RO, Wall MJ, Jr., Itani KM, et al. Chlorhexidine-Alcohol Versus Povidone-Iodine for Surgical-Site Antisepsis. *N Engl J Med* 2010;362(1):18–26. doi: 10.1056/NEJMoa0810988

2. Tuuli MG, Liu J, Stout MJ, et al. A Randomized Trial Comparing Skin Antiseptic Agents at Cesarean Delivery. *N Engl J Med* 2016;374(7):647–55. doi: 10.1056/NEJMoa1511048 [published online first: 2016/02/05]

3. Berrios-Torres SI, Umscheid CA, Bratzler DW, et al. Centers for Disease Control and Prevention Guideline for the Prevention of Surgical Site Infection, 2017. *JAMA Surg* 2017;152(8):784–91. doi: 10.1001/jamasurg.2017.0904 [published online first: 2017/05/04]

4. Yeung LL, Grewal S, Bullock A, et al. A Comparison of Chlorhexidine-Alcohol Versus Povidone-Iodine for Eliminating Skin Flora Before Genitourinary Prosthetic Surgery: A Randomized Controlled Trial. *J Urol* 2013;189(1):136–40. doi: 10.1016/j.juro.2012.08.086 [published online first: 2012/11/21]

5. O'Hara LM, Thom KA, Preas MA. Update to the Centers for Disease Control and Prevention and the Healthcare Infection Control Practices Advisory Committee Guideline for the Prevention of Surgical Site Infection (2017): A Summary, Review, and Strategies for Implementation. *Am J Infect Control* 2018;46(6):602–09. doi: 10.1016/j.ajic.2018.01.018 [published online first: 2018/03/12]

6. Ban KA, Minei JP, Laronga C, et al. Executive Summary of the American College of Surgeons/Surgical Infection Society Surgical Site Infection Guidelines—2016 Update. *Surg Infect (Larchmt)* 2017;18(4):379–82. doi: 10.1089/sur.2016.214 [published online first: 2017/05/26]

7. Levine LA, Becher EF, Bella AJ, et al. Penile Prosthesis Surgery: Current Recommendations from the International Consultation on Sexual Medicine. *J Sex Med* 2016;13(4):489–518. doi: 10.1016/j.jsxm.2016.01.017 [published online first: 2016/04/06]

8. Hebert KJ, Kohler TS. Penile Prosthesis Infection: Myths and Realities. *World J Mens Health* 2019;37(3):276–87. doi: 10.5534/wjmh.180123 [published online first: 2019/04/01]

Clean Intermittent Self-Catheterization in the Treatment of Urinary Tract Disease

JEFFREY I. ESTRIN AND SEAN P. ELLIOTT

"Patients with urinary abnormalities caused by neurogenic and atonic bladders . . . treated with a non-sterile technique of intermittent self-catheterization [showed] tremendous improvement . . . in all parameters including urinary infection . . . [which] lend[s] further support for our concept of the pathophysiology of most urinary infections."[1]

Research Question: In patients with incomplete bladder emptying, what are the outcomes of clean intermittent catherization (CIC)?

Funding: Not reported

Year Study Began: 1970

Year Study Published: 1972

Study Location: Not reported

Who Was Studied: Patients (12 female and 2 male) aged 3 to 65 years with incomplete bladder emptying due to various etiologies (multiple sclerosis, myelodysplasia, myelomeningocele, adhesive arachnoiditis, lipoma of the conus medullaris, traumatic transverse myelitis, or no discernible neurologic deficit).

Who Was Excluded: Not reported

Patients: 14

Study Overview:

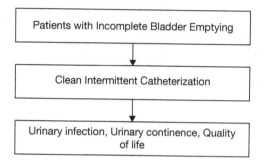

Study Interventions: Patients were taught to self-catheterize themselves after having washed their hands using a 14F plastic or rubber Robinson catheter. For small children, the mothers were taught the technique. They were also provided a water-soluble lubricant and a bottle of detergent to clean the catheters for reuse.

Follow-up: Unclear; one patient was followed for at least 6 months.

Endpoints: Urinary tract infection (UTI), urinary continence, self-reported quality of life

---

RESULTS:

- All patients were able to successfully learn and perform the technique of CIC.
- All adult patients reported that control of their urinary difficulties helped them return to "live a normal, happy life."
- The pediatric patients remained afebrile and continent, without UTIs during the study period.
- Most adult patients remained free from UTI during the study period.
- Two patients with UTI were not compliant in performing CIC at regular, frequent intervals.
- One of the patients with an atonic bladder secondary to voiding dysfunction was treated for UTI during the study.

Criticism and Limitations: The study was an uncontrolled, retrospective case series without a control group that lacked well-defined inclusion and exclusion criteria. The sample size was very small and the patient population was heterogenous, including men and women, children and adults; the patients had voiding dysfunction from a variety of neurologic and non-neurologic causes. It is not clear how closely the patients were monitored for UTI nor how UTI was defined. The study was performed before the advent of urodynamics, so the true bladder pressures are unknown. This study does not represent current practice in that it was performed before modern therapies were developed for managing bladder dysfunction. Finally, although the authors report an improvement in quality of life with the initiation of CIC, urinary quality-of-life metrics had not yet been developed.

Other Relevant Studies and Information:

- In 1976, Diokno et al. published a study of myelomeningocele patients with varying degrees of neurogenic bladder, with recurrent UTI and/or urinary incontinence.[2] Thirty-eight of 43 patients using CIC achieved satisfactory control of incontinence and a majority remained free from UTI and upper urinary tract deterioration.
- In 1981, Kass et al. evaluated children with myelomeningocele and vesicoureteral reflux (VUR) treated with CIC.[3] Reflux improved in 31% of ureters and remained stable in 24% of ureters using CIC. The remainder of patients underwent surgical reimplantation. This led to the notion of treating the bladder first when managing VUR in the setting of voiding dysfunction, thus avoiding unnecessary ureteral reimplantation, which had previously been common in such children.
- Subsequently, McGuire's group demonstrated that urodynamic findings could be used to inform management of neurogenic bladder.[4] They found that routine catheterization and anticholinergics designed to keep bladder pressures below 40 cm H_2O could significantly reduce the risk of renal damage in children with myelomeningocele.
- Kaefer et al. in 1999 evaluated the benefit of prophylactic CIC in children less than 1 year old with myelomeningocele at risk of upper tract deterioration due to detrusor–sphincter dyssynergia and/or high bladder pressures.[5] When comparing patients managed with early CIC and those managed expectantly, the CIC groups were less likely to require urinary diversion or bladder augmentation.
- Pohl et al. demonstrated the benefits of CIC in promoting continence and avoiding UTIs in the setting of dysfunctional voiding and high

postvoid residual urine volume in neurologically and anatomically normal patients.[6]

Summary and Implications: This study by Lapides et al. demonstrated the safety and efficacy of a clean, non-sterile approach to intermittent catheterization. Lapides' revolutionary idea has now become a mainstay of therapy in patients with neurogenic and non-neurogenic voiding dysfunction.[7]

CLINICAL CASE: SELF-CATHETERIZATION FOR A PATIENT WITH SPINA BIFIDA

Case History:

A 30-year-old woman with a history of sacral spina bifida voids spontaneously but has experienced increasing episodes of incontinence. Another urologist performed a mesh sling for her incontinence and her incontinence improved about 50%, but now she has urinary frequency and urinary tract infections. Cystoscopy shows a normal urethra and bladder neck with no mesh erosion. Urodynamic testing reveals an absence of detrusor overactivity but low compliance during the filling phase. Her maximum bladder capacity is 500 ml with a resting detrusor pressure of 25 cm H_2O. She leaks small volumes spontaneously at capacity. She attempts to void by Valsalva. There is no detrusor contraction. Maximum urinary flow rate is 10 ml/sec and postvoid residual is 300 ml.

Suggested Answer:

Sacral spina bifida typically presents in childhood with a weak detrusor and weak outlet. In this woman, the outlet resistance was increased by the prior sling. Because she is dependent on Valsalva voiding, she is unable to empty very well against the increased outlet resistance. Her elevated postvoid residuals may be contributing to her recurrent infections. Her incontinence is likely overflow at maximum capacity; she reaches this maximum capacity early because she empties incompletely by Valsalva, resulting in urinary frequency.

Placing her on CIC would allow her to empty completely, increasing the time between her voids. Complete emptying would also reduce her infection risk. If she catheterizes before reaching her maximum capacity, she can likely minimize her incontinence without any additional surgery.

References

1. Lapides J, Diokno AC, Silber SJ, Lowe BS. Clean, intermittent self-catheterization in the treatment of urinary tract disease. *J Urol.* 1972;107(3):458–61.
2. Diokno AC, Kass E, Lapides J. New approach to myelodysplasia. *J Urol.* 1976;116(6):771–2.
3. Kass EJ, Koff SA, Diokno AC. Fate of vesicoureteral reflux in children with neuropathic bladders managed by intermittent catheterization. *J Urol.* 1981;125(1):63–4.
4. Flood HD, Ritchey ML, Bloom DA, et al. Outcome of reflux in children with myelodysplasia managed by bladder pressure monitoring. *J Urol.* 1994;152(5 Pt 1):1574–7.
5. Kaefer M, Pabby A, Kelly M, et al. Improved bladder function after prophylactic treatment of the high risk neurogenic bladder in newborns with myelomeningocele. *J Urol.* 1999;162(3 Pt 2):1068–71.
6. Pohl HG, Bauer SB, Borer JG, et al. The outcome of voiding dysfunction managed with clean intermittent catheterization in neurologically and anatomically normal children. *BJU Int.* 2002;89(9):923–7.
7. Bloom DA, McGuire EJ, Lapides J. A brief history of urethral catheterization. *J Urol.* 1994;151(2):317–25.

The Surgical Learning Curve for Prostate Cancer Control After Radical Prostatectomy

PHILIPP DAHM

"The size of the difference in outcome associated with increasing surgical experience, and the large number of cases required before the learning curve starts to plateau, suggests that more serious attention should be paid to the issue of surgical quality."[1]

Research Question: In patients with clinically localized prostate cancer undergoing open radical prostatectomy, how does the surgeon's experience affect the risk of biochemical recurrence?

Funding: National Cancer Institute SPORE grant and philanthropic grants from the Allbritton Fund and the Koch Foundation

Year Study Began: 1987

Year Study Published: 2007

Study Location: Four major US academic medical centers (Memorial Sloan Kettering Cancer Center, Baylor College of Medicine, Wayne State University, and the Cleveland Clinic)

Who Was Studied: Men with clinically localized prostate cancer treated by open retropubic prostatectomy

Who Was Excluded: Men who received neoadjuvant therapy or adjuvant therapy or who had missed data for the treating surgeon or for the serum prostate-specific antigen (PSA) level

Patients: 7,765

Study Overview:

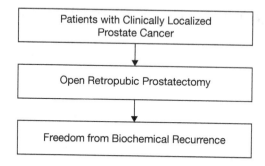

Study Interventions: All patients underwent open retropubic prostatectomy by 1 of 72 surgeons with various levels of procedure-specific experience. The relationship of surgeon experience and biochemical recurrence was modeled using a multivariable, parametric survival time regression model that accounted for within-surgeon clustering. Patients who died were censored. Model covariates were preoperative PSA level, pathological tumor stage, Gleason grade of the surgical specimen, and year of surgery (to account for stage migration).

Follow-up: Median follow-up of patients without recurrence was 3.9 years.

Endpoints: Freedom from biochemical recurrence. Biochemical recurrence was defined as a PSA level of 0.4 ng/ml followed by a subsequent higher PSA level.

RESULTS:

- There were 1,256 biochemical recurrences among 7,765 patients (16.2%).
- Most surgeons (57%) had performed fewer than 50 prostatectomies during their career to date; a substantial percentage (22%) had performed at least 100 surgeries in total (Table 50.1).
- There was dramatic improvement in cancer control with increasing surgeon experience up to 250 prior operations but no large change with further surgeon experience.

- The predicted probabilities of recurrence were 17.9% (95% confidence interval [CI], 12.1 to 25.6) for patients treated by surgeons with 10 prior surgeries and 10.7% (95% CI, 4.6 to 10.1) for patients treated by surgeons with 250 prior surgeries. This corresponds to a number needed to harm of 14.
- These results were robust to a number of sensitivity analyses, including restriction to surgery since the year 2000 as well as the addition of margin status to the model.

Table 50.1 SELECT TUMOR CHARACTERISTICS BY SURGEON EXPERIENCE

	<50	50–99	100–249	250–999	1,000 or more	p-value
Number of patients	1,402	696	1,575	2,940	1,152	
Median preoperative PSA	7.3	6.8	7.3	6.6	6.0	0.002
Extracapsular extension (%)	29.9	28.2	31.2	30.4	22.7	0.004
Seminal vesicle invasion (%)	11.7	2.5	10.5	8.5	4.5	0.001
Lymph node + (%)	4.0	4.0	3.4	4.0	3.1	0.5
5-year probability of recurrence % (95% CI)	27 (24 – 30)	23 (19 – 27)	19 (17 – 22)	16 (14 – 17)	16 (14 – 17)	

Criticism and Limitations: The major weakness of this study is that, since it was a retrospective observational study, it is possible that confounding factors explain the results. Modeling was used to adjust for differences in patients and tumor characteristics to account for confounding factors, but residual confounding is possible. In addition, this study took place at four major, high-volume academic centers and all cases involved the open retropubic approach; therefore, these findings may not apply to other populations. The only outcome assessed was the surrogate outcome of freedom of biochemical recurrence, which may not translate into disease-specific morbidity and mortality in all patients.

Other Relevant Studies and Information:

- The same lead author subsequently published a similar analysis of the surgical learning curve for laparoscopic prostatectomy.[2] The study also found that greater surgeon experience was associated with a lower risk of recurrence. The learning curve for laparoscopic radical prostatectomy was lengthier than the previously reported learning curve for open surgery. Surgeons with previous experience of open radical prostatectomy had significantly poorer results than those whose first operation was laparoscopic.

- An operative experience of 150 cases has been proposed for robotic-assisted laparoscopic prostatectomy to achieve proficiency.[3]

Summary and Implications: This study stands out as the first high-quality study in the urological literature to provide a detailed analysis of the association of surgical experience with an important clinical outcome measure with presentation of a learning curve. It provides compelling evidence that surgical experience with prostatectomy results in improved oncological outcomes. Based on these findings, patients with prostate cancer should consider choosing a high-volume surgeon.[4,5]

CLINICAL CASE: ROBOTIC-ASSISTED LAPAROSCOPIC VERSUS OPEN RETROPUBIC PROSTATECTOMY

Case History:

A 54-year-old patient in a rural part of the country is diagnosed with cT2 Gleason score 4 + 4 (5 of 12 cores bilaterally; PSA 12.5 ng/ml) high-risk prostate cancer. A bone scan and computed tomography scan demonstrate no evidence of metastatic disease. After discussing treatment options both with his urologist and a radiation oncologist, he elects to undergo radical prostatectomy and bilateral pelvic lymph node dissection. His urologist does not perform robotic surgery but reports a personal experience of over 500 open retropubic prostatectomies over the last 15 years; in the last year alone, he performed 45 cases. The patient also sees an advertisement by another hospital in his vicinity that has recently acquired the Da Vinci robotic surgery. When seeking a second opinion about surgery there, another urologist assures him that he has completed all the necessary training required by the manufacturer and that an experienced proctor would be on hand to oversee all aspects of the case. However, he remains vague on his actual surgical experience.

Suggested Answer:

Neither American Urological Association[6] nor European Association of Urology guidelines[7] recommend a specific surgical approach, but the latter specifically speaks to the role of experience and careful attention to detail in order to improve surgical cancer control. The proven benefit of a robotic-assisted approach relates to a reduced risk of transfusion and shorter length of stay, whereas oncological and functional outcomes are probably similar in experienced hands.[6,8] Therefore, surgical experience should outweigh surgical experience. The fact that the urologist offering to perform robotic-assisted surgery would be operating with oversight by a proctor would suggest that he remains in his early learning curve (he has likely performed fewer than 10 cases). Given that the patient has the alternative choice of a surgeon who is experienced in performing open surgery, he should probably choose the latter.

References

1. Vickers AJ, Bianco FJ, Serio AM, et al. The surgical learning curve for prostate cancer control after radical prostatectomy. *J Natl Cancer Inst* 2007;99(15):1171–7. doi: 10.1093/jnci/djm060

2. Vickers AJ, Savage CJ, Hruza M, et al. The surgical learning curve for laparoscopic radical prostatectomy: a retrospective cohort study. *Lancet Oncol* 2009;10(5):475–80. doi: 10.1016/S1470-2045(09)70079-8 [published online first: 2009/04/04]

3. Herrell SD, Smith JA, Jr. Robotic-assisted laparoscopic prostatectomy: what is the learning curve? *Urology* 2005;66(5 Suppl):105–7. doi: 10.1016/j.urology.2005.06.084 [published online first: 2005/10/01]

4. Begg CB, Scardino PT. Taking stock of volume-outcome studies. *J Clin Oncol* 2003;21(3):393–4. doi: 10.1200/JCO.2003.11.022 [published online first: 2003/02/01]

5. Lipscomb J. Transcending the volume-outcome relationship in cancer care. *J Natl Cancer Inst* 2006;98(3):151–4. doi: 10.1093/jnci/djj055 [published online first: 2006/02/02]

6. Sanda MG, Cadeddu JA, Kirkby E, et al. Clinically localized prostate cancer: AUA/ASTRO/SUO guideline. Part II: recommended approaches and details of specific care options. *J Urol* 2018;199(4):990–7. doi: 10.1016/j.juro.2018.01.002 [published online first: 2018/01/15]

7. Mottet N, Bellmunt J, Bolla M, et al. EAU-ESTRO-SIOG guidelines on prostate cancer. Part 1: screening, diagnosis, and local treatment with curative intent. *Eur Urol* 2017;71(4):618–29. doi: 10.1016/j.eururo.2016.08.003 [published online first: 2016/08/30]

8. Ilic D, Evans SM, Allan CA, et al. Laparoscopic and robotic-assisted versus open radical prostatectomy for the treatment of localised prostate cancer. *Cochrane Database Syst Rev* 2017;9:CD009625. doi: 10.1002/14651858.CD009625.pub2 [published online first: 2017/09/13]

INDEX

Tables are indicated by *t* following the page number

Abbott Laboratories, 269
ABC (Anticholinergic Versus Botulinum Toxin Comparison) Study, 239–43
abiraterone, in prostate cancer, 95–99
active monitoring, in prostate cancer, 43–47
active surveillance, in prostate cancer, 25–30, 40
ADT. *See* androgen deprivation therapy
Advanced Bladder Cancer Meta-analysis Collaboration, 143–44
alcohol: chlorhexidine–alcohol scrub, 275–79, 277*t*
Allbritton Fund, 287
alpha-blockers, in BPH, 269–74, 271*t*
alprostadil, transurethral: for ED, 251–55
American College of Physicians: guidelines for ureteral stones, 186
American College of Surgeons: recommendations for surgical-site antisepsis, 278
American Kidney Fund, 189
American Urological Association (AUA)
    active surveillance recommendations, 28, 40
    bladder cancer guidelines, 131
    female SUI guidelines, 235
    kidney stone guidelines, 191, 199–200
    male LUTS attributable to BPH guidelines, 272
    midurethral sling recommendations, 224
    prostate cancer guidelines, 28, 34, 40, 52, 58, 97, 290–91
    radical prostatectomy recommendations, 34
    renal cell carcinoma guidelines, 110
    stress incontinence guidelines, 218
    ureteral stone guidelines, 186, 209
    VUR prevention guidelines, 260–61
    watchful waiting recommendations, 22
androgen blockade, in prostate cancer, 76
androgen deprivation therapy (ADT)
    clinical case, 80
    intermittent, 77–81
    in prostate cancer, 64, 67–71, 77–81
anticholinergic therapy: for urgency incontinence, 239–43
Anticholinergic Versus Botulinum Toxin Comparison (ABC) Study, 239–43
antimicrobial prophylaxis: for VUR, 257–61
antisepsis, surgical-site: methods for, 275–79, 277*t*
ARO 96-02 trial, 64
Association Française Genitourinary Group (GETUG-AFU)-15 study, 91
Astellas Pharma, 101
AstraZeneca, 77
Australian Public Health Service, 153
autologous fascia pubovaginal sling: vs. Burch colposuspension, 218
Aventis Pharma (now Sanofi), 83

avodart: Combination of Avodart and
Tamsulosin (CombAT) study, 272

bacillus Calmette–Guérin (BCG): for
bladder cancer, 135–39
Baylor College of Medicine, 287
Beckman Coulter, 1
benign prostatic hyperplasia (BPH)
LUTS attributed to, 266–67
with moderate symptoms, 263–68
surgery vs. watchful waiting for, 263–68
terazosin and finasteride for, 269–74,
271t
BEP (cisplatin, etoposide, and bleomycin)
for germ cell tumors, 177–81
for poor-risk non-seminoma, 180
biopsy
MRI-guided, 13–17
transrectal ultrasound-guided (TRUS),
13–17
bladder cancer
advanced, 159–63
BCG for, 135–39
bladder-preserving multimodality
therapy for, 150
chemotherapy for, 141–45, 147–51
cystectomy +/- chemotherapy for,
141–45
GC vs. M-VAC in, 159–63
guidelines for, 131, 144, 149–50
locally advanced, 141–45
metastatic, 159–63
MMC for, 129–33
muscle-invasive, 147–51
radiotherapy in, 147–51
recurrent, 129–33, 135–39
superficial, 129–33
transitional cell carcinoma, 135–39
transurethral resection of, 132
urothelial, 138
bleomycin
cis-diamminedichloroplatinum,
vinblastine, and bleomycin
combination chemotherapy, 171–75
cisplatin, etoposide, and bleomycin
(BEP), 177–81

cisplatin, vinblastine, and bleomycin
(PVB), 177–81
in disseminated germ cell tumors,
177–81
in disseminated testicular cancer, 171–75
in poor-risk non-seminoma, 180
Boston Scientific, 197
Botox (onabotulinumtoxin A): for
urgency incontinence, 239–43
brachytherapy: quality of life after, 55–59,
57t
Bristol-Myers Squibb, 123
Burch colposuspension: for stress
incontinence, 215–19

calcium stones
dietary calcium and, 189–92
water intake and, 183–87
Cancer and Leukemia Group B, 141
Cancer Center, 177
Cancer du Rein Metastatique
Nephrectomie et Antiangiogéniques
(CARMENA) trial, 115
Cancer of the Prostate Strategic Urologic
Endeavor (CaPSURE) registry, 69
Cancer Research UK, 147
CAP (Cluster Randomized Trial of PSA
Testing), 45
CaPSURE (Cancer of the Prostate
Strategic Urologic Endeavor)
registry, 69
Cardinal Health, 275–76
CARE (Colpopexy and Urinary
Reduction Efforts) trial, 229
CARMENA (Cancer du Rein
Metastatique Nephrectomie et
Antiangiogéniques) trial, 115
catheterization: self-catheterization,
281–85
Centers for Disease Control and Prevention
(CDC): recommendations for
surgical-site antisepsis, 278
CHAARTED (Chemohormonal
Therapy Versus Androgen Ablation
Randomized Trial for Extensive Disease
in Prostate Cancer) Trial, 86, 89–93

CheckMate 025, 123–27
CheckMate 214, 125
chemohormonal therapy, in prostate cancer, 89–93
Chemohormonal Therapy Versus Androgen Ablation Randomized Trial for Extensive Disease in Prostate Cancer (CHAARTED) Trial, 86, 89–93
chemotherapy. See also specific drugs
  for bladder cancer, 141–45
  cisplatinum-based, 174
  combination, 171–75
  cystectomy +/-, 141–45
  docetaxel-based, 92, 98
  enzalutamide before, in metastatic prostate cancer, 101–5
  for poor-risk non-seminoma, 180
  for prostate cancer, 83–87, 85t, 89–93, 101–5
  radiation +/-, 141–45
  for testicular cancer, 171–75
  for urothelial carcinoma, 156
children: antimicrobial prophylaxis for VUR, 257–61
ChloraPrep (Cardinal Health), 276
chlorhexidine–alcohol scrub: for surgical-site antisepsis, 275–79, 277t
CIC (clean intermittent catheterization), 281–85
cisplatin
  in bladder cancer, 141–45, 159–63
  cis-diamminedichloroplatinum, vinblastine, and bleomycin combination chemotherapy, 171–75
  cisplatin, etoposide, and bleomycin (BEP), 177–81
  cisplatin, vinblastine, and bleomycin (PVB), 177–81
  gemcitabine and cisplatin (GC), 159–63
  in germ cell tumors, 177–81
  methotrexate, vinblastine, doxorubicin, and cisplatin (M-VAC), 141–45, 153–57, 159–63
  in non-seminoma, 180

  in testicular cancer, 171–75
  in urothelial carcinoma, 153–57
clean intermittent catheterization (CIC), 281–85
Cleveland Clinic, 287
Cluster Randomized Trial of PSA Testing (CAP), 45
colic, ureteric: MET for, 209–13
Colpopexy and Urinary Reduction Efforts (CARE) trial, 229
colposuspension, Burch: for stress incontinence, 215–19
Combination of Avodart and Tamsulosin (CombAT) study, 272
Cougar Biotechnology, 95
cystectomy +/- chemotherapy: for bladder cancer, 141–45

dietary calcium: and kidney stones, 189–92
dietary counseling: for prevention of calcium stones, 192
docetaxel
  abiraterone after, 98
  for prostate cancer, 83–87, 85t, 92
doxorubicin
  in bladder cancer, 141–45, 159–63
  methotrexate, vinblastine, doxorubicin, and cisplatin (M-VAC), 141–45, 153–57, 159–63
  in urothelial carcinoma, 153–57

Eastern Cooperative Oncology Group (ECOG), 141
EAU. See European Association of Urology
ECOG (Eastern Cooperative Oncology Group), 141
ED. See erectile dysfunction
Eli Lilly and Company, 159
enzalutamide, in prostate cancer, 101–5
EORTC. See European Organisation for Research and Treatment of Cancer
erectile dysfunction (ED)
  sildenafil for, 245–49, 247t
  transurethral alprostadil for, 251–55

ERSPC (European Randomized Study of Screening for Prostate Cancer), 1–5
ESMO. *See* European Society of Medical Oncology
ESWL. *See* extracorporeal shock wave lithotripsy
etoposide
cisplatin, etoposide, and bleomycin (BEP), 177–81
in disseminated germ cell tumors, 177–81
in poor-risk non-seminoma, 180
Europe Against Cancer, 1
European Association of Urology (EAU)
active surveillance recommendations, 28, 40
bladder cancer guidelines, 131, 144, 149–50
female SUI guidelines, 235–36
kidney stone guidelines, 191, 199–200
male LUTS attributable to BPH guidelines, 272
midurethral sling recommendations, 224
MRI-guided biopsy recommendations, 16
prostate cancer guidelines, 34, 52, 58, 80, 97, 290–91
renal cell carcinoma guidelines, 110, 116
stress incontinence guidelines, 218
ureteral stone guidelines, 186, 209
watchful waiting recommendations, 22
European Organisation for Research and Treatment of Cancer (EORTC)
Intergroup Phase 3 Study comparing elective nephron-sparing surgery and radical nephrectomy for low-stage renal cell carcinoma, 107–11
trial 22911, 64
European Randomized Study of Screening for Prostate Cancer (ERSPC), 1–5
European Society of Medical Oncology (ESMO): guidelines for second-line therapy for metastatic RCC, 126

European Union, 1
everolimus, in advanced RCC, 123–27
external-beam radiotherapy (EBRT): quality of life after, 55–59, 57t
extracorporeal shock wave lithotripsy (ESWL)
first clinical experience, 193–96
for kidney stones, 193–96
for lower-pole kidney stones, 197–201, 203–7
vs. ureteroscopy, 197–201

fascial slings: for stress incontinence, 215–19
finasteride
adverse effects, 271, 271t
combined with terazosin, 269–74, 271t
effects in BPH, 269–74, 271t
effects in prostate cancer, 7–11
flutamide: orchiectomy with or without, 73–76
Food and Drug Administration (FDA): safety warnings about PDE-5 inhibitors, 9
Foods Cancer (FOCA), 77, 107

gemcitabine and cisplatin (GC), in bladder cancer, 159–63
Genitourinary Group of the Association Françoise (GETUG-AFU)-15 study, 91
German Ministry of Research and Technology, 193
germ cell tumors: BEP vs. PVB for, 177–81
GETUG-AFU (Genitourinary Group of the Association Françoise)-15 study, 91

Health Professionals Follow-Up Study, 185
hormone-sensitive prostate cancer
chemohormonal therapy for, 89–93
docetaxel-based chemotherapy for, 92
metastatic, 89–93

IAD. *See* intermittent androgen deprivation

IFN. *See* interferon

Immediate Surgery or Surgery After Sunitinib Malate in Treating Patients with Kidney Cancer (SURTIME) trial, 115–16

immunotherapy
   BCG, 135–39
   for bladder cancer, 135–39

Indiana University Medical Center, 171

infection
   antimicrobial prophylaxis for VUR, 257–61
   surgical-site, 275–79, 277t

inflatable penile prosthesis (IPP) surgery, 278

interferon
   IFN +/- nephrectomy, for metastatic RCC, 113–17
   vs. sunitinib, in metastatic RCC, 119–22

intermittent androgen deprivation (IAD)
   clinical case, 80
   in prostate cancer, 77–81

International Consultation on Sexual Medicine, 278

intraurethral alprostadil: for ED, 254

iodine: povidone–iodine scrub, 275–79, 277t

IPP (inflatable penile prosthesis) surgery, 278

KEYNOTE-045, 165–69

KEYNOTE-057, 168

kidney stones
   calcium stones, 183–87
   dietary calcium and, 189–92
   ESWL for, 193–96, 203–7
   guideline recommendations for treatment of, 199–200
   large, 203–7
   lower-pole, 197–201, 203–7
   percutaneous nephrolithotomy for, 203–7
   shock wave lithotripsy for, 197–201
   small, 197–201
   symptomatic, 189–92

ureteroscopy for, 197–201
   water intake and, 183–87

Koch Foundation, 287

laparoscopic surgery. *See* robotic-assisted laparoscopic prostatectomy (RALP)

lithotripsy. *See* extracorporeal shock wave lithotripsy (ESWL)

Lower Pole I Study, 195, 203–7

lower-pole kidney stones
   ESWL for, 197–201, 203–7
   PCNL for, 203–7
   treatment of, 203–7

lower urinary tract symptoms (LUTS)
   guideline recommendations for, 272
   terazosin, finasteride, or both in, 269–74, 271t
   TURP in, 266–67

magnetic resonance imaging (MRI)
   -guided biopsy for prostate cancer diagnosis, 13–17
   multiparametric, 16–17

Massachusetts Male Aging Study, 253

medical expulsive therapy (MET): for ureteral colic, 209–13

Medical Research Council (UK), 129

Medical Therapy of Prostatic Symptoms (MTOPS) study, 272

Medivation, 101

Memorial Sloan Kettering Cancer Center, 287

Merck and Co., 165, 269

MET (medical expulsive therapy): for ureteral colic, 209–13

metabolic stone management: guideline recommendations for, 191

metastatic bladder cancer: GC vs. M-VAC in, 159–63

metastatic prostate cancer
   abiraterone effects in, 95–99
   androgen blockade in, 76
   chemohormonal therapy for, 89–93
   enzalutamide in, 101–5
   hormone-sensitive, 89–93
   orchiectomy with or without flutamide in, 73–76

metastatic renal cell carcinoma
  first-line treatment of, 122
  IFN +/- nephrectomy for, 113–17
  nivolumab vs. everolimus in, 123–27
  second-line treatment of, 126
  sunitinib vs. IFN in, 119–22
metastatic urothelial carcinoma
  cisplatin vs. M-VAC in, 153–57
  GC vs. M-VAC in, 159–63
methotrexate, vinblastine, doxorubicin,
    and cisplatin (M-VAC)
  in bladder cancer, 141–45, 159–63
  in urothelial carcinoma, 153–57
Microvasive, 203
midurethral slings
  for incontinence, 221–25
  preoperative evaluation before surgery,
    236–37
  retropubic vs. transobturator, 221–25
  vaginal prolapse repair and, 227–31
minimally invasive radical prostatectomy
    (MIRP): vs. retropubic
    prostatectomy, 49–54, 51t
mitomycin C (MMC): for bladder cancer,
    129–33
mitoxantrone: for prostate cancer, 83–87,
    85t
MMC (mitomycin C): for bladder cancer,
    129–33
monitoring, active: in prostate cancer,
    43–47
MRI. See magnetic resonance imaging
MTOPS (Medical Therapy of Prostatic
    Symptoms) study, 272
M-VAC. See methotrexate, vinblastine,
    doxorubicin, and cisplatin

National Cancer Institute (NCI) (US),
    61, 67, 73, 77, 89, 107, 113, 135,
    141, 153, 287
  Public Health Service grants, 7
National Cancer Institute of Canada, 61,
    153
National Comprehensive Cancer
    Network (NCCN) (US): guidelines
    for bladder cancer, 144

National Health Service (UK), 209
National Institute for Health and Care
    Excellence (NICE)
  SUI guidelines, 236–37
  vaginal prolapse repair
    recommendations, 230
National Institute for Health Research
    (UK), 43, 147, 209
National Institute of Child Health and
    Human Development (NICHD)
    (US), 215, 221, 227, 233, 239
National Institute of Diabetes and Digestive
    and Kidney Diseases (NIDDK) (US),
    215, 221, 227, 233, 257
National Institutes of Health (NIH) (US),
    55, 177, 189
  Office of Research in Women's Health
    (ORWH), 215, 227, 239
nephrectomy
  cytoreductive, 116
  IFN +/-, for metastatic RCC, 113–17
  radical, 107–11
nephrolithiasis. See kidney stones
nephrolithotomy, percutaneous, 203–7
nephron-sparing surgery (NSS): vs.
    radical nephrectomy, 107–11
nivolumab: vs. everolimus, in advanced
    RCC, 123–27
NSS (nephron-sparing surgery): vs.
    radical nephrectomy, 107–11
Nurses' Health Study I, 185, 191
Nurses' Health Study II, 191
nutrients, dietary: and kidney stones,
    189–92

observation
  in prostate cancer, 31–35, 37–42,
    61–66, 63t
  vs. prostatectomy, 1–5, 31–35, 37–42
onabotulinumtoxin A (Botox): for
    urgency incontinence, 239–43
open retropubic prostatectomy
  vs. minimally invasive prostatectomy,
    49–54
  vs. robotic-assisted laparoscopic
    surgery (RALP), 53, 290–91

OPUS (Outcomes Following Vaginal Prolapse Repair and Midurethral Sling) Trial, 227–31

orchiectomy: with or without flutamide, 73–76

Outcomes Following Vaginal Prolapse Repair and Midurethral Sling (OPUS) Trial, 227–31

PCNL (percutaneous nephrolithotomy): for lower-pole kidney stones, 203–7

PCOS (Prostate Cancer Outcomes Study), 58

PCPT (Prostate Cancer Prevention Trial), 7–11

Pelvic Floor Disorders Network (PFDN), 227

pembrolizumab, in urothelial cancer, 165–69

percutaneous nephrolithotomy (PCNL): for lower-pole kidney stones, 203–7

PFDN (Pelvic Floor Disorders Network), 227

Pfizer, 119, 245

PIVOT (Prostate Cancer Intervention Versus Observation Trial), 22, 28, 34, 37–42, 39t

PLCO (Prostate, Lung, Colon, and Ovarian) Cancer Screening Trial, 3

povidone–iodine scrub: for surgical-site antisepsis, 275–79, 277t

PRECISION trial, 13–17

prednisone: for prostate cancer, 83–87

PREVAIL Study, 101–5

Prevention of Recurrent Urinary Tract Infection in Children with Vesicoureteric Reflux and Normal Renal Tracts (PRIVENT) trial, 259

Prostate, Lung, Colon, and Ovarian (PLCO) Cancer Screening Trial, 3

prostate cancer
10-year outcomes, 43–47
abiraterone effects in, 95–99
active surveillance for, 25–30, 40
advanced, 61–66, 63t, 83–87, 85t

androgen deprivation therapy for, 64, 67–71, 77–81

bilateral orchiectomy with or without flutamide in, 73–76

chemohormonal therapy for, 89–93

chemotherapy for, 83–87, 85t

conservative management of, 19–23

early, 31–35

enzalutamide in, 101–5

finasteride effects in, 7–11

guidelines for treatment of, 58

hormone-sensitive, 89–93

localized, 1–5, 19–23, 25–35, 37–47, 49–54, 51t, 55–59, 57t, 67–71

low-grade, 19–23

low-risk, 10, 28–29

metastatic, 73–76, 89–93, 95–99, 101–5

monitoring, 43–47

MRI-guided diagnosis of, 13–17

quality of life after primary treatment, 55–59, 57t

after radical prostatectomy, 287–91, 289t

radiotherapy for, 43–47, 55–59, 57t, 61–66, 63t

screening for, 1–5

surgery for, 43–47

watchful waiting in, 19–23

Prostate Cancer Intervention Versus Observation Trial (PIVOT), 22, 28, 34, 37–42, 39t

Prostate Cancer Outcomes Study (PCOS), 58

Prostate Cancer Prevention Trial (PCPT), 7–11

prostatectomy
minimally invasive vs. open, 49–54, 51t
vs. observation, 31–35, 37–42
in prostate cancer, 1–5, 31–35, 37–42, 49–54, 51t
prostate cancer control after, 287–91, 289t
quality of life after, 55–59, 57t
radical, 1–5, 31–35, 37–42, 49–54, 51t, 55–59, 57t, 287–91, 289t
robotic-assisted laparoscopic vs. open retropubic, 52–53, 290–91

prostate-specific antigen (PSA) screening
    clinical case, 4, 16–17
    Cluster Randomized Trial of PSA
        Testing (CAP), 45
    multiparametric MRI for, 16–17
    vs. no screening, 1–5
Prostate Testing for Cancer and
    Treatment (ProtecT) Trial, 28, 34,
    43–47, 58
prostatic hyperplasia. See benign prostatic
    hyperplasia (BPH)
ProtecT (Prostate Testing for Cancer and
    Treatment) Trial, 28, 34, 43–47, 58
PSA screening. See prostate-specific
    antigen (PSA) screening
pubovaginal slings: vs. Burch
    colposuspension, 218
PVB (cisplatin, vinblastine, and
    bleomycin): for germ cell tumors,
    177–81

quality of life: after primary prostate
    cancer treatment, 55–59, 57t

Radiation Therapy and Androgen
    Deprivation Therapy in Treating
    Patients Who Have Undergone
    Surgery for Prostate Cancer
    (RADICALS-RT) trial, 64
radical nephrectomy: vs. nephron-sparing
    surgery (NSS), 107–11
radical prostatectomy
    minimally invasive (MIRP), 49–54, 51t
    vs. observation, 1–5, 31–35, 37–42
    in prostate cancer, 1–5, 31–35, 37–47,
        49–54, 51t
    prostate cancer control after, 287–91,
        289t
    quality of life after, 55–59, 57t
    vs. radiotherapy and active monitoring,
        43–47
    vs. robotic-assisted laparoscopic
        surgery (RALP), 53
radical retropubic prostatectomy (RRP)
    in localized prostate cancer, 49–54, 51t
    vs. minimally invasive, 49–54, 51t

    vs. robotic-assisted laparoscopic
        surgery (RALP), 52–53
    RADICALS-RT (Radiation Therapy and
        Androgen Deprivation Therapy
        in Treating Patients Who Have
        Undergone Surgery for Prostate
        Cancer) trial, 64
radiotherapy
    for bladder cancer, 147–51
    with chemotherapy, 147–51
    external-beam (EBRT), 55–59, 57t
    for prostate cancer, 43–47, 55–59, 57t,
        61–66, 63t
    quality of life after, 55–59, 57t
RALP. See robotic-assisted laparoscopic
    prostatectomy
Randomized Intervention for Children
    With Vesicoureteral Reflux
    (RIVUR) Trial, 257–61
RCC. See renal cell carcinoma
REDUCE trial, 9
reflux, vesicoureteral (VUR): antimicrobial
    prophylaxis for, 257–61
renal cell carcinoma
    advanced, 123–27
    first-line treatment of, 122
    guidelines for, 110
    IFN +/- nephrectomy for, 113–17
    low-stage, 107–11
    metastatic, 113–17, 119–27
    nivolumab vs. everolimus in, 123–27
    sunitinib vs. interferon alfa in, 119–22
renal masses, small: treatment of, 110
renal stones. See kidney stones
retropubic midurethral slings: for stress
    incontinence, 221–25
retropubic prostatectomy, open
    vs. minimally invasive, 49–54
    vs. robotic-assisted laparoscopic
        surgery (RALP), 53, 290–91
RIVUR (Randomized Intervention
    for Children With Vesicoureteral
    Reflux) Trial, 257–61
robotic-assisted laparoscopic
    prostatectomy (RALP)
    clinical case, 53

vs. open retropubic prostatectomy, 52–53, 290–91

RRP. See radical retropubic prostatectomy

Sanofi, 83, 89

Scandinavian Prostate Cancer Group Trial 4 (SPCG-4), 21, 31–35, 40

screening: for prostate cancer, 1–5, 16–17

Scrub Care Skin Prep Tray (Cardinal Health), 276

SELECT trial, 10

self-catheterization, 281–85

shock wave lithotripsy (SWL)
  extracorporeal (ESWL), 193–201, 203–7
  for kidney stones, 193–96
  for lower-pole renal stones, 197–201, 203–7
  vs. ureteroscopy, 197–201

sildenafil: for ED, 245–49, 247t

SISTEr (Stress Incontinence Surgical Treatment Efficacy) Trial, 215–19

slings
  fascial, 215–19
  for incontinence, 215–19, 221–25
  midurethral, 221–25, 227–31, 236–37
  prophylactic surgery with, 230
  vaginal prolapse repair and, 227–31

Society of Urodynamics, Female Pelvic Medicine and Urogenital Reconstruction (SUFU): guideline recommendations for female SUI, 235

Southwest Oncology Group (SWOG), 73, 113, 136, 141
  Trial 8794 (SWOG 8794), 61–66, 63t
  Trial 9346 (SWOG 9346), 77–81
  Trial 9916 (SWOG 9916), 85

SPCG-4 (Scandinavian Prostate Cancer Group Trial 4), 21, 31–35, 40

spina bifida, 284

Spontaneous Urinary Stone Passage Enabled by Drugs (SUSPEND) Trial, 209–13

STAMPEDE (Systemic Therapy in Advancing or Metastatic Prostate Cancer: Evaluation of Drug Efficacy), 86, 91

START (Surveillance Therapy Against Radical Treatment) trial, 27

stones. See also kidney stones
  calcium, 189–92
  metabolic management of, 191
  urinary, 209–13

Stress Incontinence Surgical Treatment Efficacy (SISTEr) Trial, 215–19

stress urinary incontinence (SUI)
  Burch colposuspension vs. fascial sling for, 215–19
  guideline recommendations, 235–37
  midurethral slings for, 221–25
  surgery for, 215–19
  urodynamic tests before surgery, 233–37

SUFU (Society of Urodynamics, Female Pelvic Medicine and Urogenital Reconstruction): guideline recommendations for female SUI, 235

SUI. See stress urinary incontinence

sulfamethoxazole: trimethoprim-sulfamethoxazole (TMP-SMX), 257–61

sunitinib
  vs. IFN, in metastatic RCC, 119–22
  Immediate Surgery or Surgery After Sunitinib Malate in Treating Patients with Kidney Cancer (SURTIME) trial, 115–16

surgery. See also specific procedures
  for BPH, 263–68, 265t
  incontinence, 215–19, 233–37
  inflatable penile prosthesis (IPP), 278
  laparoscopic, 52–53
  midurethral sling, 236–37
  nephron-sparing (NSS), 107–11
  for prostate cancer, 43–47
  for renal cell carcinoma, 107–11
  sling, 230
  transurethral resection of prostate (TURP), 263–68
  urodynamic tests before, 233–37
  vaginal prolapse repair, 227–31

surgical learning curve, 287–91, 289t

surgical-site antisepsis: methods for, 275–79, 277t
SURTIME (Immediate Surgery or Surgery After Sunitinib Malate in Treating Patients with Kidney Cancer) trial, 115–16
surveillance
    active, 25–30, 40
    for prostate cancer, 25–30, 40
Surveillance Therapy Against Radical Treatment (START) trial, 27
SUSPEND (Spontaneous Urinary Stone Passage Enabled by Drugs) Trial, 209–13
Swedish Cancer Society, 31
SWL. See shock wave lithotripsy
SWOG. See Southwest Oncology Group
Systemic Therapy in Advancing or Metastatic Prostate Cancer: Evaluation of Drug Efficacy (STAMPEDE), 86, 91

tadalafil: for ED, 248
tamsulosin: Combination of Avodart and Tamsulosin (CombAT) study, 272
TAX 327 Trial, 83–87, 85t
terazosin
    adverse effects, 271, 271t
    combined with finasteride, 269–74, 271t
    effects in BPH, 269–74, 271t
testicular cancer: combination chemotherapy in, 171–75
TMP-SMX (trimethoprim-sulfamethoxazole), in preventing UTI recurrence, 257–61
TOMUS (Trial of Mid Urethral Slings), 221–25
transitional cell carcinoma of bladder: BCG for, 135–39
transobturator midurethral slings: for stress incontinence, 221–25
transrectal ultrasound-guided (TRUS) biopsy: for prostate cancer diagnosis, 13–17
transurethral alprostadil: for ED, 251–55

transurethral bladder cancer resection: intravesical MMC after, 132
transurethral resection of prostate (TURP): for BPH, 263–68, 265t
Trial of Mid Urethral Slings (TOMUS), 221–25
trimethoprim–sulfamethoxazole (TMP-SMX), in preventing UTI recurrence, 257–61
TRUS (transrectal ultrasound-guided) biopsy: for prostate cancer diagnosis, 13–17

UCC. See urothelial cell carcinoma
UDS (urodynamic studies): before incontinence surgery, 233–37
UITN (Urinary Incontinence Treatment Network), 216, 221, 233
University of Munich, Germany, 193
University of Parma, Italy, 183
ureteral stones: secondary prevention of, 186
ureteric colic: MET for, 209–13
ureteroscopy (URS): for lower-pole kidney stones, 197–201
urgency urinary incontinence (UUI): Botox for, 239–43
urinary incontinence
    Botox for, 239–43
    Burch colposuspension vs. fascial sling for, 215–19
    midurethral slings for, 221–25, 227–31
    stress, 215–19, 221–25, 233–37
    urgency, 239–43
    after vaginal prolapse repair, 227–31
Urinary Incontinence Treatment Network (UITN), 216, 221, 233
urinary stones: Spontaneous Urinary Stone Passage Enabled by Drugs (SUSPEND) Trial, 209–13
urinary tract disease: clean intermittent catheterization (CIC) treatment of, 281–85
urinary tract infection (UTI): antimicrobial prophylaxis for VUR, 257–61

urinary volume: and kidney stones, 183–87

urodynamic studies (UDS): before incontinence surgery, 233–37

urothelial cell carcinoma (UCC)
advanced, 156, 159–63, 165–69
cisplatin vs. M-VAC in, 153–57
GC vs. M-VAC in, 159–63
metastatic, 153–57, 159–63
pembrolizumab in, 165–69

URS. *See* ureteroscopy

US Department of Defense Prostate Cancer Physician Training Award, 49

US Department of Health and Human Services, 141

US Department of Veterans Affairs Cooperative Studies Program, 37, 263, 269

US Preventive Services Task Force: recommendation against PSA screening, 4

UTI (urinary tract infection): antimicrobial prophylaxis for VUR, 257–61

UUI (urgency urinary incontinence): Botox for, 239–43

vaginal prolapse repair: and midurethral slings, 227–31

Value of Urodynamic Evaluation (ValUE) Trial, 233–37

vesicoureteral reflux (VUR): antimicrobial prophylaxis for, 257–61

Veterans Affairs Cooperative Benign Prostatic Hyperplasia Study, 269–74

Veterans Affairs Cooperative Study Group on Transurethral Resection of the Prostate, 263–68

Veterans Affairs Medical Centers, 263, 269

vinblastine
in bladder cancer, 141–45, 159–63
cis-diamminedichloroplatinum, vinblastine, and bleomycin combination chemotherapy, 171–75
cisplatin, vinblastine, and bleomycin (PVB), 177–81
in disseminated germ cell tumors, 177–81
in disseminated testicular cancer, 171–75
methotrexate, vinblastine, doxorubicin, and cisplatin (M-VAC), 141–45, 153–57, 159–63
in urothelial carcinoma, 153–57

Vivus, Inc., 251

VUR (vesicoureteral reflux): antimicrobial prophylaxis for, 257–61

watchful waiting
in BPH, 263–68, 265t
in prostate cancer, 19–23

water intake: and kidney stones, 183–87

Wayne State University, 287